THE METABOLIC SYNDROME
AND YOUR HEART

THE NEW
GLUCOSE
revolution

Other books in the New Glucose Revolution Series

THE METABOLIC SYNDROME AND YOUR HEART

THE NEW GLUCOSE *revolution*

KAYE FOSTER-POWELL
PROF JENNIE BRAND-MILLER
DR ANTHONY LEEDS

HODDER

A Hodder Book

First published in Australia and New Zealand in 1999 as
The GI Factor: The Glucose Revolution Your Heart
by Hodder Headline Australia Pty Limited
(A member of the Hodder Headline Group)
Level 22, 201 Kent Street, Sydney NSW 2000
Website: www. hha. com. au

Reprinted 2000
Published as *The New Glucose Revolution Your Heart*
in 2002

This edition published as the *New Glucose Revolution The Metabolic Syndrome and Your Heart* in 2003

National Library of Australia Cataloguing-in-Publication

Brand Miller, Jennie, 1952- .
  The metabolic syndrome & your heart : the new glucose
  revolution.

  ISBN 0 7336 1650 X.

  1. Glycemic index. 2. Food – Carbohydrate content. 3. Heart –
  Diseases – Prevention. 4. Diet therapy – Recipes. I. Leeds,
  Anthony R. II. Foster-Powell, Kaye. III. Brand Miller, Jennie,
  1952- The new glucose revolution : your heart. IV. Title.

613.283

Cover by Greendot Design
Cover image © photolibrary. com
Typeset by Egan-Reid Ltd, Auckland
Printed in Australia by Griffin Press, Adelaide

CONTENTS

INTRODUCTION

Did you know that heart disease is the single biggest killer of Australians? Every 10 minutes, every day, someone in Australia suffers a cardiovascular event. So what causes this deadly disease? Often it is a result of atherosclerosis or 'hardening of the arteries'. We now know it's not just a 'plumbing' problem, but one in which inflammation plays a key role.

Heart disease, however, seldom occurs as an isolated condition. One in two Australians over 25 years of age has at least two features of the 'silent' disease: the metabolic syndrome (sometimes called the insulin resistance syndrome or Syndrome X). The metabolic syndrome is a collection of metabolic abnormalities—like a 'pot belly', high blood pressure, high blood glucose, low levels of 'good' cholesterol—that increase your risk of atherosclerosis and heart attack.

While most people these days are aware of the importance of cutting back on fat to minimise our risk of heart disease, very few people are aware that the type of carbohydrate we eat can also help prevent heart disease and improve the metabolic syndrome.

Research on the glycemic index of foods, what we have called the GI, shows that the type of carbohydrate we eat may have as much influence on our risk of heart disease as the type of fat we eat.

As we explain in our bestselling book, *The New Glucose Revolution*, the glycemic index:

- is a scientifically proven measure of the effect carbohydrates have on blood glucose levels;
- helps you choose the right amount and type of carbohydrate for your health and wellbeing;
- provides an easy and effective way to eat a healthy diet and control fluctuations in blood glucose.

It's vital that people learn about the GI so they base their diet on sound scientific evidence.

What is the GI?

The glycemic index (GI) is a physiologically based measure of carbohydrate quality—a comparison of carbohydrates (gram for gram) based on their immediate effect on blood glucose levels.

- Carbohydrates that break down quickly during digestion have **high GI** values. Their blood glucose response is fast and high.
- Carbohydrates that break down slowly, releasing glucose gradually into the blood stream, have a **low GI**.

The rate of carbohydrate digestion has important implications for everybody. For more detailed information about the glycemic index and its many benefits you should consult *The New Glucose Revolution* or *The New Glucose Revolution Life Plan*.

THE METABOLIC SYNDROME AND YOUR HEART

WHAT THIS BOOK CAN DO FOR YOU

Understanding the GI has made an enormous difference to the diet and lifestyle of many people. Recent studies show that diets rich in slowly digested carbohydrates with a low glycemic index:

- reduce blood cholesterol levels
- reduce the 'bad' LDL cholesterol
- increase the 'good' HDL cholesterol
- reduce CRP (a measure of chronic, low-grade inflammation)
- increase the body's sensitivity to insulin
- improve blood flow
- reduce hunger
- help weight control

In practical terms this means that:

- our intake of bread, potatoes, rice and pasta can influence our risk of heart disease
- a diet rich in quickly digested carbohydrates may increase our risk of a heart attack
- eating more fruit, wholegrains, dried peas and beans and low fat dairy foods can reduce our risk of heart disease

In this book we will show you how vitally important an understanding of the GI is for your heart health and how easy it is to make the change to a low GI diet. We will:

- explain how the GI is measured
- outline the beneficial aspects of the GI for heart health
- show you how to include more of the right sort of carbohydrate in your diet
- give practical hints to help you make the GI work for you throughout the day
- provide a week of low GI menus with nutritional analysis
- list the GI of over 400 foods for easy reference

UNDERSTANDING THE GLYCEMIC INDEX

The glycemic index concept was first developed in 1981 by Dr. David Jenkins, a professor of nutrition at the University of Toronto, Canada, to help determine which carbohydrates were best for people with diabetes. At that time, the diet for people with diabetes was based on a system of carbohydrate exchanges, which assumed that all starchy foods produced the same effect on blood glucose levels, even though earlier studies had already proven this was not correct. Jenkins was one of the first people to question this assumption and investigate how real foods behave in the bodies of real people.

Since then, scientists, including the authors of this book, have tested the effect of different foods on blood glucose levels and other biochemical factors. Clinical studies in the United Kingdom, France, Italy, Australia and Canada all have proven without doubt the value of the glycemic index.

The GI of foods is simply a ranking of carbohydrates in foods according to their immediate impact on blood glucose levels. To make a fair comparison, all foods are compared with a reference food such as pure glucose and are tested in equivalent carbohydrate amounts.

Today we know the GI of hundreds of different food items that have been tested following the standardised method. We have included many of these values in the tables at the back of this book, but for more detailed information you should consult *The New Glucose Revolution* or *The New Glucose Revolution Complete Guide to GI Values*.

The key is the rate of digestion

Foods containing carbohydrates that break down quickly during digestion have the highest GI value. The blood glucose response is fast and high (in other words, the glucose in the bloodstream increases rapidly). Conversely, foods that contain carbohydrates which break down slowly, releasing glucose gradually into the bloodstream, have low GI values.

For most people, the foods with a low GI have advantages over those with high GI values. This is especially true for those people trying to prevent the metabolic syndrome and atherosclerosis.

The higher the GI, the higher the blood glucose levels after consumption of the food. Instant white rice (GI of 87) and baked potatoes (GI of 85) have very high GIs, meaning their effect on blood glucose levels is almost as high as that of an equal amount of pure glucose (yes, you read it correctly).

Low GI = 55 or less
Intermediate GI = 56 to 69
High GI = 70 or more

Figure 1 shows the blood glucose response to potatoes compared with pure glucose. Foods with a low GI (like lentils at 29) show a flatter blood glucose response when eaten, as shown in Figure 2. The peak blood glucose level is lower and the return to baseline levels is slower than with a high GI food.

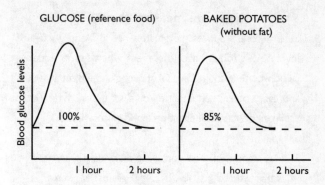

Figure 1. The effect of pure glucose (50 g) and baked potatoes without fat (50 g carbohydrate portion) on blood glucose levels.

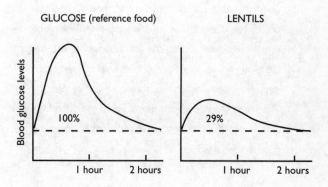

Figure 2. The effect of pure glucose (50 g) and lentils (50 g carbohydrate portion) on blood glucose levels.

How we measure the GI

Pure glucose produces the greatest rise in blood glucose levels. Most foods have less effect when fed in equal carbohydrate quantities. The GI of pure glucose is set at 100 and every other food is ranked on a scale from 1 to 100 according to its actual effect on blood glucose levels.

1. An amount of food containing a standard amount of carbohydrate (usually 25 or 50 grams) is given to a volunteer to eat. For example, to test boiled spaghetti, the volunteer will be given 200 grams of spaghetti which supplies 50 grams of carbohydrate (determined from food composition tables).

2. Over the next two hours (or three hours if the volunteer has diabetes), we take a sample of their blood every 15 minutes during the first hour and thereafter every 30 minutes. The blood glucose level of these blood samples is measured in the laboratory and recorded.

3. The blood glucose level is plotted on a graph and the area under the curve is calculated using a computer program (Figure 3).

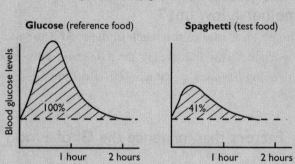

Figure 3. Measuring the GI of a food

The test food and the reference food must contain the same amount of carbohydrate. The usual dose is 50 grams but sometimes 25 grams is used when the portion size would be otherwise too large. Even smaller doses such as 15 grams have been used. The GI result is much the same whatever the dose because the GI is simply a relative measure of carbohydrate quality.

4. The volunteer's response to spaghetti (or whatever food is being tested) is compared with his or her blood glucose response to 50 grams of pure glucose (the reference food).

5. The reference food is tested on two or three separate occasions and an average value is calculated. This is done to reduce the effect of day-to-day variation in blood glucose responses.

6. The average GI found in 8–10 people is the GI of that food.

What gives one food a high GI and another a low one?

The physical state of the starch in the food is the most important factor influencing the GI. That's why food processing has such a profound effect on the GI.

Factors that influence the GI of a food

Factor	Mechanism	Examples of food where the effect is seen
Starch gelatinisation	The less gelatinised (swollen) the starch, the slower the rate of digestion.	Spaghetti, porridge, biscuits have less gelatinised starch.
Physical entrapment	The fibrous coat around beans and seeds and plant cell walls acts as a physical barrier, slowing down access of enzymes to the starch inside.	Pumpernickel and grainy bread, legumes and barley.
High amylose to amylopectin ratio*	The more amylose a food contains, the less easily the starch is gelatinised and the slower its rate of digestion.	Basmati rice, legumes, and Hi-Maize™ starch contain more amylose than other cereals.
Particle size	The smaller the particle size, the easier it is for water and enzymes to penetrate (the surface area is relatively higher).	Finely milled flours have high GIs. Stone-ground flours have larger particles and lower GIs.

Factors that influence the GI of a food *(cont.)*

Factor	Mechanism	Examples of food where the effect is seen
Viscosity of fibre	Viscous, soluble fibres increase the viscosity of the intestinal contents and this slows down the interaction between the starch and the enzymes. Finely milled wholemeal wheat and rye flours have fast rates of digestion and absorption because the fibre is not viscous.	Rolled oats, beans and lentils, apples, Metamucil®.
Sugar	The digestion of sugar produces only half as many glucose molecules as the same amount of starch (the other half is fructose). The presence of sugar also restricts gelatinisation of the starch by binding water and reducing the amount of 'available' water.	Some biscuits, some breakfast cereals that are high in sugar have relatively low GI values.
Acidity	Acids in foods slow down stomach emptying, thereby slowing the rate at which the starch can be digested.	Vinegar, lemon juice, lime juice, salad dressings, pickled vegetables, sourdough bread.
Fat	Fat slows down the rate of stomach emptying, thereby slowing the digestion of the starch.	Potato crisps have a lower GI than boiled potatoes.

* Amylose and amylopectin are two different types of starch. Both are found in foods, but the ratio varies.

WHAT IS HEART DISEASE?

As we mentioned earlier most heart disease is caused by atherosclerosis of the arteries, sometimes referred to as 'hardening of the arteries'. Generally, people develop atherosclerosis gradually during their lifetime and live much of their life blissfully unaware of it. If it develops fairly slowly it may not cause any problems, even into great old age, but if its development is accelerated by one or more of many processes (such as high cholesterol or high glucose levels) the condition may cause trouble much earlier in life.

Atherosclerosis

Atherosclerosis results in reduced blood flow through the affected arteries. In the heart this can mean that the heart muscle gets insufficient oxygen to provide the power for pumping blood and it changes in such a way that pain is experienced (central chest pain or angina pectoris). Elsewhere in the body, atherosclerosis has a similar blood flow reducing effect: in the legs it can cause muscle pains on exercise; in the brain it can cause a variety of problems from 'funny turns' to strokes;

An even more serious consequence of atherosclerosis occurs when a blood clot forms over the surface of a patch of atherosclerosis on an artery. This process of thrombosis can result in a complete blockage of the artery, with consequences ranging from sudden death to a small heart attack from which the patient generally recovers quickly.

The process of thrombosis can occur elsewhere in the arterial system with outcomes determined by the extent of the thrombosis. The probability of developing thrombosis is determined by the 'tendency' of the blood to clot versus the natural ability of the blood to break down clots (fibrinolysis). These two counteracting 'tendencies' are influenced by a number of factors, including the level of glucose in the blood.

Knowing your blood glucose level is just as
important as knowing your cholesterol level.

People who have gradually developed atherosclerosis of
the arteries to the heart (the coronary arteries) may
slowly develop reduced heart function. For a while the
heart may be able to compensate for the problem, so
there are no symptoms, but eventually it begins to fail.
Shortness of breath may occur, initially on exercise, and
sometimes there may be some swelling of the ankles.
Atherosclerosis can also lead to abnormal heart beat
(palpitations).

Modern medicine has many effective drug
treatments for heart failure so this consequence of
atherosclerosis does not have quite the same serious
implications as it did in the past.

Why do people get heart disease?

For most people atherosclerotic heart disease develops early in life when the many factors that cause it have a strong influence. Over many decades doctors and scientists have identified the processes which cause heart disease in fine detail and now most of the factors are well known.

Theoretically, atherosclerotic heart disease might be largely prevented if everyone's risks were assessed in youth and if all the right things were done throughout the rest of their lives. In practice, there has been limited development of the ways to screen people for risk early in life, and the resources needed to achieve prevention are just not available.

A great deal is already being done, however, to identify risk factors (i.e. 'red flags') in healthy people and those with established heart disease. A high cholesterol level is a well-established risk factor, as is a low level of HDL—the 'good' cholesterol.

More recently, high glucose levels after eating have been shown to be an important, but under-recognised predictor of both cardiovascular disease and death from any cause. High levels of glucose in the blood, even transient increases such as after a meal, have many undesirable effects, stemming from the fact that glucose increases the production of 'free radicals'. Free radicals are highly reactive, charged molecules that inflict harm on everything close by. They damage proteins, fats and cellular structures. In particular, they cause inflammation of the cells lining blood vessels. We now recognise that atherosclerosis is an inflammatory disease.

The good news is that those of us who take the necessary action will reduce our risk.

We discuss the risk factors for heart disease further on pages 28–34.

High glucose levels after eating have been shown to be an important predictor or cardiovascular disease. A low GI diet helps reduce post-meal blood glucose levels.

HOW CAN THE GI HELP?

The type of carbohydrate we eat determines the body's blood glucose response and also determines the levels of insulin in our blood for many hours after eating. High insulin levels caused by eating foods with a high GI are undesirable. In the long term, they promote high blood fat, high blood glucose, high blood pressure and increase the risk of heart attack.

Because of this, the GI of the diet is significant in the long-term prevention of heart disease and may be equally important in the diets of people who already have heart disease.

Firstly, a low GI diet has benefits for weight control, helping to satisfy appetite and preventing overeating and excessive body weight.

Secondly, it helps reduce post-meal blood glucose levels in both normal and diabetic individuals. This improves the elasticity of the walls of the arteries, making dilation easier and improving blood flow.

Thirdly, blood fats and clotting factors can be improved by low GI diets.

Low GI diets also reduce total blood cholesterol and low-density (LDL) cholesterol in people with undesirably high levels. Lower levels of total cholesterol and LDL cholesterol are associated with a lower risk of heart disease.

Specifically, population studies have shown that HDL cholesterol levels are correlated with the GI and glycemic load of the diet. Those of us who self-select the lowest GI diets have the highest and best levels of HDL—the good cholesterol.

HDL cholesterol is a sign of cholesterol being taken away from arteries, so the higher the levels the better. Large scale surveys have shown that high HDL cholesterol is the best predictor of a lower risk of heart disease. One of the key features of the metabolic syndrome is a low HDL level.

Furthermore, research studies in people with diabetes have shown that low GI diets reduce triglycerides in the blood, a factor strongly linked to the metabolic syndrome. Lastly, low GI diets have been shown to improve insulin sensitivity in people at high risk of heart disease, thereby helping to reduce the rise in blood glucose and insulin levels after normal meals.

By working on several fronts at one time, low GI diets have a distinct advantage over other types of diets or drugs that target only one risk factor at a time.

One study in particular has provided the best evidence in support of the role of the GI in heart disease. The study was conducted by Harvard University and is commonly referred to as 'the Nurses Study'. The Nurses Study is an ongoing, long-term study of over 100 000 nurses who provide their personal health and diet information to researchers at Harvard School of Public Health every few years. In this way, diet can be linked with the future development of different diseases. It found that those who ate more high GI foods had nearly twice the risk of having a heart attack over a ten-year period of follow-up, compared to those eating low GI diets. This association was independent of dietary fibre and other known risk factors, such as age and body mass index. In other words, even if fibre intake was high, there was still an adverse effect of high GI diets on risk. Importantly, neither sugar nor total carbohydrate intake showed any association with risk of heart attack. Thus there was no evidence that lower carbohydrate or sugar intake was helpful.

One of the most important findings of the Nurses Study was that the increased risk associated with high GI diets was largely seen in those with a body mass index (BMI) over 23 (to calculate your body mass divide your weight in kilograms by the square of your height in metres). There was no increased risk in those under 23. But the fact remains that the great majority of adults have a BMI greater than 23; indeed a BMI of 23–25 is considered normal weight. The implication therefore is that the insulin resistance that comes with increasing weight is an integral part of the disease process. So, if you are very lean and insulin sensitive, high GI diets won't make you more prone to heart attack. This might explain why traditional-living Asian populations, such as the Chinese, who eat high GI rice as a staple food, do not show increased risk of heart disease. Their low BMI and their high level of physical activity conspire to keep them insulin sensitive and extremely carbohydrate tolerant.

> The GI may reduce the risk of heart disease by increasing the 'good' cholesterol and reducing the level of triglycerides (fats) in the blood.

Treating the metabolic syndrome and heart disease

When the metabolic syndrome or actual signs of heart disease are detected two types of treatment are given. Firstly, the effects of the disease are treated (e.g. medical treatment with drugs and surgical treatment to bypass blocked arteries) and, secondly, the risk factors are treated to slow down further progression of the disease.

Treatment of risk factors after the disease has already developed is 'secondary prevention'. In people who have not yet developed the disease (e.g. those with insulin resistance), treatment of risk factors is 'primary prevention'.

Obviously it would be better to give primary preventive treatment in all cases but the GI has application in both cases.

Preventing heart disease

More and more people now get regular checks of their blood pressure, and tests to check for diabetes. Increasingly, blood cholesterol tests are done to check this risk factor too. If your medical practitioner is on the ball, he or she will also do a blood glucose test.

All health professionals give lifestyle advice on stopping smoking, the benefits of exercise and the nature of a good diet. When specific risk factors are discovered, diet and lifestyle advice is given, but sometimes may not be followed for long.

It is especially difficult to follow advice if the effect of not following it is likely not to matter for ten or more years, and if the changes needed are not attractive. The changes must be wanted by the individual who will be helped by encouragement from friends and relatives, and the changes must ideally be positive changes—'I want to do this', not 'They've told me to do this.'

TEST YOUR HEART KNOWLEDGE

Try this quick quiz on diet and heart disease to test your knowledge. Answer true or false to the following:

1. All vegetable oils are low in saturated fat.
2. Butter contains more fat than margarine.
3. Australians eat more fat now than 10 years ago.
4. Eggs should be avoided on a low fat, cholesterol-lowering diet.
5. Moderate consumption of alcohol increases your risk of heart attack.
6. Olive oil has the lowest fat content of any oil.
7. A cup of milk contains less fat than two squares of chocolate.
8. Nuts will raise cholesterol levels.
9. Potato and pasta are fattening foods.
10. Cod liver oil will lower cholesterol levels.

The answer to each of the preceding questions is false. Here's an explanation why ...

1. Contrary to popular belief, not all vegetable oils are low in saturated fat. Two primary exceptions are coconut oil and palm or palm kernel oil. Both these oils (which may appear on a food label simply as vegetable oil) are highly saturated. Palm oil is used widely in commercial cakes, biscuits, pastries and fried foods.

2. Butter and margarine contain similar levels of fat (around 85–90 per cent). There is a difference in the types of fats which predominate, however, butter being about 60 per cent saturated fat and unsaturated margarines being less than 30 per cent saturated fat.

3. Australians are eating less fat now than 10 years ago. In 1988, we ate 35 per cent of our energy in the form of fat. Now we are down to 32 per cent but we still have a way to go to achieve 30 per cent. Plus, these are average figures, so many of us are still eating far too much fat.

4. Eggs are a source of cholesterol but dietary cholesterol tends to raise blood cholesterol levels only when the background diet is high in fat. One egg contains only about 5 grams of fat, of which only 2 grams is saturated.

5. Moderate amounts of alcohol (e.g. 2 standard drinks per day) appear to reduce the risk of heart attack. Amounts in excess are harmful to health.

6. There is no such thing as low fat oil. Oil is fat in a liquid form, its fat content being 100 per cent. Olive oil is a suitable choice of oils containing only 15 per cent saturated fats. Mediterranean populations, whose major source of fat is olive oil, have low levels of heart disease.

7. A cup (250 ml) of full cream milk contains 10 grams of fat. Compare this to about four grams contained in two small squares of chocolate!

8. Nuts have been found to be protective against heart disease. While most nuts are high in fat, much of the fat they contain is of the 'good' unsaturated types.

9. This myth has been around for years. Potato and pasta are high carbohydrate foods which means they are a good source of energy for the body. They are rarely stored as body fat.

10. Cod liver oil has not been found to lower cholesterol levels. It is extremely rich in vitamins A and D and should not be taken in large doses because of the danger of vitamin A toxicity.

HEART DISEASE RISK FACTORS

Your chance of developing heart disease is increased if you smoke tobacco, have high blood pressure, have diabetes or 'pre-diabetes' (high glucose levels but not yet as high as in diabetes), have high blood cholesterol (which may be due to eating too much saturated fat in your diet), are overweight or obese and/or sedentary.

Low saturated fat and low GI
help prevent heart disease.

Smoking

Smoking tobacco is now clearly established as a cause of atherosclerosis. Few authorities dispute the evidence. There are, however, some interesting dietary aspects. Did you know that:

- smokers tend to eat less fruit and vegetables compared to non-smokers (and thus eat less of the protective anti-oxidant plant compounds); and
- smokers tend to eat more fat and more salt than non-smokers?

These characteristics of the smoker's diet may be caused by a desire to seek strong food flavours as a consequence of the taste-blunting effect of smoking. While these dietary differences may make the smoker at greater risk of heart disease there is only one piece of advice for anyone who smokes:

Please stop smoking!

High blood pressure

High blood pressure (hypertension) is very damaging because it demands that your heart work harder and it damages your arteries. Remember, an artery is not a rigid pipe, it is a muscular tube, which when healthy can change its size to control the flow of blood.

High blood pressure causes changes in the walls of arteries which makes atherosclerosis more likely to develop. Blood clots can then form and the weakened blood vessels can easily thrombose or rupture and bleed. In Australia, approximately 1 in 2 people aged 65 years and over is hypertensive.

Treatments for blood pressure have become more effective over the last thirty years, but it is only now becoming clear which types of treatment for blood pressure are also effective at reducing heart disease risk.

Normal range for blood pressure: less than 140/90 mm Hg

Diabetes and 'pre-diabetes'

Diabetes is, in itself, a further risk factor for heart disease. Diabetes is caused by a lack of insulin—either the body does not produce enough, or the body 'demands' more than normal (because it has become insensitive to insulin). Diabetes and pre-diabetes (impaired glucose tolerance) cause inflammation and hardening of the arteries. When glucose levels are raised, even temporarily (such as after eating), oxidising reactions are accelerated and the level of anti-oxidants such as vitamin E and C decline. In particular, the blood fats are oxidised, making them more damaging to artery walls. The walls become inflamed, thicken and gradually lose their elasticity. The constriction of the arteries results in increased blood pressure. If that's not bad enough, high insulin levels increase the tendency for blood clots to form. The resulting increased risk of heart attack is a major reason why we put so much effort into helping people with diabetes achieve normal control of blood glucose and also why all people with diabetes should be checked for the other risk factors of heart disease. But you don't need to have diabetes to be at risk—even moderately raised blood glucose levels hours after a meal have been associated with increased risk of heart disease in normal 'healthy' people.

High cholesterol

High blood cholesterol also increases your risk of heart disease. Your blood cholesterol is determined by genetic (inherited) factors, which you cannot change, and lifestyle factors, which you can change.

There are some relatively rare genetic conditions in which particularly high blood cholesterol levels occur. People who have inherited these conditions need a thorough examination by a specialist doctor followed by life-long drug treatment.

In most people, high blood cholesterol is partly determined by their genes, which have 'set' the cholesterol level slightly high, and lifestyle factors which push it up more. Body weight also affects blood cholesterol—in some people, being overweight has a significant effect on the levels, so attaining a reasonable weight can be helpful. The most important dietary factor is fat, in particular, saturated fat. Diets recommended for blood cholesterol lowering are low fat (particularly saturated fat), high carbohydrate, high fibre diets.

The blood also contains triglycerides, another type of fat which may be linked with increased risk of heart disease in some people. Levels of both cholesterol and triglyceride need to be checked as part of an assessment of your risk of heart disease.

High cholesterol foods?

Many people who aim to lower their risk of heart disease focus on avoiding foods that are high in cholesterol. But this is putting the emphasis in the wrong place. Cholesterol itself is concentrated in very few foods (see below) and is not the main cause of our high blood cholesterol levels. In fact, the amount of cholesterol we obtain from food is generally much less than the amount of cholesterol our body makes. Our body can make all the cholesterol we need, but in certain circumstances, our body makes more cholesterol than necessary. This causes the level of cholesterol in our blood to build up and become a problem.

Very few foods are high in cholesterol. Those which are include:

- Brains, liver and kidney
- Egg yolk
- Caviar

A diet high in saturated fat is the biggest contributor to high blood cholesterol. Reducing saturated fat intake can usually improve cholesterol levels.

CRP (C-reactive protein)

CRP in the blood is a new and powerful risk factor for heart disease. It is a measure of chronic low grade inflammation, indicative of the damaging effect of high glucose levels and other factors on the blood vessel walls. In women, it predicts future risk of heart disease better than cholesterol levels. Together, CRP and your cholesterol level are a new way for doctors to sort out those at greater risk.

Studies from Harvard have shown that the level of CRP is higher in women ingesting high GI/high glycemic load diets. That's one more good reason to choose low GI!

Normal ranges for:	
Cholesterol	< 5.2 mmol/L
Triglycerides	1.0–2.3 mmol/L
HDL cholesterol	1.0–2.5 mmol/L
Total cholesterol/HLD ratio	< 4.5
Fasting glucose	3.5–6.0 mmol/L
Non-fasting glucose	< 11.1
Glycated haemoglobin	3.5–6.0%
Insulin	< 80 pmol/L

OBESITY AND HEART DISEASE

Overweight and obese people are more likely to have high blood pressure and to have diabetes. They are also at increased risk of developing heart disease. Some of that increased risk is due to the high blood pressure, and the tendency to diabetes, but there is a separate 'independent' effect of the obesity.

Two in three Australian men are
overweight or obese.
Half of Australian women are
overweight or obese.

When increased fatness develops it can be distributed evenly all over the body or it may occur centrally—in and around the abdomen (tummy)—a 'pot belly'. This form of obesity is strongly associated with heart disease. In fact, you can have a pot belly and still be normal weight. But that extra fat around the middle is playing havoc with your metabolism. Every effort should be made to achieve and maintain a reasonable body weight —especially if your extra weight is 'middle-age spread'

How's your shape?

Fat around the middle part of our body (abdominal fat) increases our risk of heart disease, high blood pressure and diabetes. In contrast, fat on the lower part of the body, such as hips and thighs, doesn't carry the same health risk. Your body shape can be described according to your distribution of body fat as either an 'apple' or a 'pear' shape.

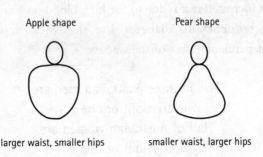

Apple shape

Pear shape

larger waist, smaller hips

smaller waist, larger hips

There are significant health benefits in reducing your waist measurement, particularly if you can have an 'apple' shape.

You can easily tell if you are an 'apple' or a 'pear' by placing a tape measure around your waist and then your hips and seeing which is smaller. Ideally the waist is smaller than the hips. If it isn't, you're an apple!

Specifically, the waist measurement for people 19 years and over should be:

- less than 102 cm for men;
- less than 88 cm for women;

If you are overweight, or consider yourself over-weight, chances are that you have looked at countless books, brochures and magazines offering a solution to losing weight. New diets or miracle weight loss solutions seem to appear weekly. They are clearly good for selling magazines, but for the majority of people who are over-weight the 'diets' don't work—if they did, there wouldn't be so many!

At best—while you stick to it—a 'diet' will reduce your kilojoule intake. At its worst, a 'diet' will change your body composition for the fatter. This is because many diets employ the technique of drastically reducing your carbohydrate intake to bring about quick weight loss. The weight you lose, however, is mostly water (that was trapped or held with stored carbohydrate) and muscle (as it is broken down to produce the glucose you need to fuel your brain). Once you return to your former way of eating, your body contains a little less muscle mass. With each repetition of a diet you lose more muscle.

Not all foods are equal. When it comes to losing weight, it is not necessarily a matter of reducing how much you eat. Research has shown that the type of food you give your body determines what it is going to burn and what it is going to store as body fat. It has also revealed that certain foods are more satisfying to the appetite than others.

This is where the GI plays a leading role. Low GI foods have two essential advantages for people trying to lose weight:

1. They fill you up and keep you satisfied for longer.

2. They help you burn more body fat and less muscle.

What's wrong with a low carbohydrate diet?

There is little scientific evidence to back up or refute low carbohydrate diets. One reason for the popularity of low carbohydrate diets for weight loss is that initial loss is rapid. Within the first few days, the scales will be reading two to three kilograms lower—the trouble is that most of that weight loss isn't body fat, but muscle glycogen and water.

When carbohydrate is no longer being supplied in sufficient amounts by your diet, the body uses its small carbohydrate reserves to fuel muscle contraction. One gram of carbohydrate in the form of muscle and liver glycogen binds four grams of water. So when you use up your total reserves of 500 grams of glycogen within the first few days, you also lose two kilograms of water, for a total loss of 2.5 kilograms, none of it fat. Conversely, when you return to normal eating, the carbohydrate reserves will be rapidly replenished along with the water.

People who have followed low carbohydrate diets for any length of time observe that the rate of weight loss plateaus off and they begin to feel rather tired and lethargic. That's not surprising because the muscles have little in the way of glycogen stores. Strenuous exercise requires both fat and carbohydrate in the fuel mix. So, in the long term, these low carbohydrate diets may discourage people from the physical exercise patterns that will help them keep their weight under control.

Our advice is that the best diet for weight control is one you can stick to for life—one that includes your favourite foods and which accommodates your cultural and ethnic heritage. Choosing low GI foods will not only promote weight control, it will reduce postprandial glycemia, increase satiety, provide bulk and a rich supply of micronutrients.

Only low GI diets have the weight of scientific evidence in their favour.

Eating to lose weight with low GI foods is easier because you don't have to go hungry, you get to eat your favourite foods, and what you end up with is true fat release.

EXERCISE—WE CAN'T LIVE WITHOUT IT!

These days it is increasingly easy to overeat. Refined foods, convenience foods and fast foods frequently lack fibre and conceal fat so that before we feel full, we have overdosed on kilojoules.

It is even easier not to exercise. With intake exceeding output on a regular basis, the result for too many of us is a lounge lizard lifestyle and subsequent weight gain.

Why exercise keeps you moving

The effect of exercise doesn't stop when you stop moving. People who exercise have higher metabolic rates and their bodies burn more kilojoules per minute even when they are asleep!

How exercise helps

Regular physical activity can reduce our blood glucose
levels, lower our risk of heart and blood vessel disease,
lower high blood pressure, increase stamina, reduce stress
and help us relax. It is meant for us all.

- Exercise speeds up our metabolic rate. By increasing
  our kilojoule expenditure, exercise helps to balance
  our sometimes excessive kilojoule intake from food
  and helps us control our weight.
- Exercise makes our muscles better at using fat as a
  source of fuel. By improving the way insulin works,
  exercise increases the amount of fat we burn.

A low GI diet has the same effect. Low GI foods reduce
the amount of insulin we need, which makes fat easier
to burn and harder to store. Since body fat is what you
want to get rid of when you lose weight, exercise in
combination with a low GI diet makes a lot of sense!

Remember that reduction in body weight takes
time. Even after you've made changes in your exercise
habits your weight may not be any different on the scales
(this is particularly true in women whose bodies tend
to gain muscle and lose fat at the same time). So don't
weigh yourself obsessively—use a tape measure around
the waist instead.

So what can you do?

We need to adapt our lifestyle to our more kilojoule-laden diet and fewer physical demands. It's important to catch bursts of physical activity whenever we can to increase our energy output.

Your increased movement may be planned, for example, walking 20 to 30 minutes 6 to 7 days a week. Home-based walking programs like this seem to be one of the best strategies for increasing physical output. Team up with a friend.

Besides planned activity you simply need to move around more in your day. Some suggestions:

- Never use a lift or an escalator if you can help it!
- Read a magazine on a stationary bike
- Coast on a treadmill while you watch the news or talk on the telephone
- Hide the remote control
- Walk to the corner shops
- Dance with your kids
- Park a hundred metres or more from work
- Take the dog for a walk

Personal trainers can improve adherence to an exercise program, if you are willing to pay for the privilege of being regularly motivated by someone with appropriate skills.

Whatever it takes for you, do it. Regard movement as an opportunity to improve your mental and physical well-being and not an inconvenience.

Cardiovascular fitness

Cardiovascular fitness is improved by regular strenuous exercise so that the blood supply to the heart may be 'improved'. Specifically, cardiovascular fitness is improved by exercise which is aerobic. This means activity that makes your heart beat faster so your pulse increases and you breathe more deeply.

Current thinking has it that we need to accumulate at least 30 minutes each day of this level of exertion to maintain cardiovascular fitness. Exercise is also important in maintaining body weight and has effects on metabolism and some factors related to blood clotting.

Getting regular exercise is clearly important. So don't just think about it, just do it!

How to make your exercise successful

Some key factors to make exercise successful include:

- seeing a benefit for yourself (e.g. your clothes fit)
- enjoying what you do
- feeling that you can do it fairly well
- fitting in with your daily life
- being inexpensive and accessible

THE GI AND THE METABOLIC SYNDROME

Surveys show that 1 in 2 Australian adults over 25 years of age has at least two features of what is seen to be a silent disease: the metabolic syndrome, or insulin resistance syndrome. This syndrome (sometimes called syndrome X) is a collection of metabolic abnormalities that 'silently' increase your risk of heart attack. The list of features is getting longer and longer, and the number of diseases linked to insulin resistance is growing.

The metabolic syndrome is set to be the disease of the early 21st century.
One in two adults are likely to suffer from the debilitating effects of this condition.

Insulin resistance

In this condition the body is insensitive, or 'partially deaf', to insulin. The organs and tissues that ought to respond to even a small rise in insulin remain unresponsive. The body tries harder by secreting more insulin to achieve the same effect, just as you might raise your voice or shout for a hard-of-hearing person. Thus high insulin levels are part and parcel of insulin resistance. Tests on patients with the metabolic syndrome show that insulin resistance is very common.

You probably have insulin resistance if you have two or more of the following:

- high blood pressure
- 'pre-diabetes'
- low HDL-cholesterol levels
- high waist circumference
- high uric acid levels in blood
- fasting glucose greater than 6 millimoles per litre
- post-glucose load greater than 7.8 millimoles per litre
- high triglycerides

Chances are your total cholesterol levels are within the normal range, giving you and your doctor a false impression of your coronary health.

You might also be normal weight (or overweight) but your waist circumference is high (more than 90 cm in women, more than 100 cm in men), indicating excessive fat around the abdomen.

But the red flag is that your blood glucose and insulin levels after a glucose load, or after eating, remain high. Resistance to the action of insulin is thought to underlie and unite all the features of this cluster of metabolic abnormalities.

One of the questions that's often asked is why insulin resistance is so common. We know that both genes and environment play a role. People of Asian, Indian or Australian Aboriginal origins appear to be more insulin resistant than those of European extraction, even when they are still young and lean.

But regardless of ethnic background, insulin resistance develops as we age. This has been attributed not to age per se, but to the fact that as we get older, we gain excessive fat around our middle, we become less physically active and we lose some of our muscle mass. It's also likely that diet plays a role—high fat diets have been associated with insulin resistance; high carbohydrate diets with improving insulin sensitivity.

Insulin resistance as we age results in the metabolic syndrome and gradually lays the foundations of a heart attack and other diseases (stroke, polycystic ovarian syndrome, fatty liver, acne, cognitive impairment).

How can the GI help?

Can a low GI diet help? In a recent study, patients with serious disease of the coronary arteries were given either low or high GI diets before surgery for coronary bypass grafts. They were given blood tests before their diets and just before surgery, and at surgery small pieces of fat tissue were removed for testing.

The tests on the fat showed that the low GI diets made the tissues of these 'insulin insensitive' patients more sensitive—in fact they were back in the same range as normal 'control' patients after just a few weeks on the low GI diet.

If people with serious heart disease can be improved would the same happen with younger people? In another study, young women in their thirties were divided into those who did and those who did not have a family history of heart disease. They themselves had not yet developed the condition. They had blood tests followed by low or high GI diets for four weeks, after which they had more blood tests, and then when they had surgery (for conditions unrelated to heart disease) pieces of fat were again removed and tested for insulin sensitivity. The young women with a family history of heart disease were insensitive to insulin originally (those without the family history of heart disease were normal) but after four weeks on the low GI diet their insulin sensitivity was back within the normal range.

In both studies the diets were designed to try to ensure that all the other variables (total energy, total carbohydrates) were not different, so that the change in insulin sensitivity was likely to have been due to the low GI diet rather than any other factor.

**Research strongly suggests
low GI diets improve the sensitivity
of the body to insulin.**

Polycystic ovarian syndrome (PCOS)

Polycystic ovarian syndrome occurs in women when multiple cysts form on the ovaries during the menstrual cycle and interfere with normal ovulation. Acne and facial hair are part of the problem, as well as being overweight, especially around the middle. PCOS is often diagnosed when women have irregular periods or find it difficult to fall pregnant.

It is now known that insulin resistance is often severe in women with PCOS and that any means of improving insulin sensitivity (drugs, weight loss) will improve outcomes. Some physicians have found that low GI diets are particularly useful for women with PCOS but, at present, there is little research to back this up. However, since low GI diets will help reduce weight and have been shown to improve insulin sensitivity in individuals at risk of coronary heart disease, it makes a lot of sense to try the low GI approach.

Low GI diets

Work on these exciting findings continues but what is known so far strongly suggests that low GI diets not only improve blood glucose in people with and without diabetes, but also the sensitivity of the body to insulin. It will take many years of further research to show that this simple dietary change will definitely slow the progress of atherosclerosis. In the meantime it is clear that risk factors for heart disease are improved by the low GI diet.

Low GI diets are consistent with the other required dietary changes needed for prevention of heart disease: they are bulky; filling; high in micronutrients, anti-oxidants and good fats; and help weight control.

Low saturated fat + low GI =
Prevention of heart disease

HOW DOES YOUR DIET RATE?

Reducing the GI of your diet will reduce insulin levels and increase the potential for fat burning. You can achieve an effective reduction in the GI by substituting a least one high GI carbohydrate choice at each meal with a low GI food. It's the carbohydrate foods that you eat the most of which have the greatest impact—so check your intake using the following table.

You don't have to avoid all
high GI foods to eat a low GI diet.
Try and eat one low GI food per meal.

What type of carbohydrate did you eat yesterday?

1. Recall the carbohydrate-rich foods that you ate yesterday. Remember to think of snacks as well as the main meals!
2. Tick the check boxes below for the types of foods you ate.

High GI	Low GI

Starchy foods

☐ Potato, including baked, mashed, steamed, boiled and chips
☐ Rice (Calrose, arborio, Sunbrown Quick, instant rice, jasmine)

Starchy foods

☐ Sweet corn
☐ Baked beans
☐ Sweet potato
☐ Chickpeas
☐ Kidney beans, lentils
☐ Pasta
☐ Noodles
☐ Basmati or Doongara rice

Bread Products

☐ White bread
☐ Wholemeal bread
☐ Crumpets
☐ Pikelets
☐ Scones
☐ Bagels
☐ French bread

Bread Products

☐ Wholegrain bread
☐ Fruit loaf, raisin toast
☐ Sourdough bread
☐ Performax
☐ Burgen Soy-Lin, Rye or Oat-bran and Honey

High GI	Low GI

Cereals

- ☐ Cornflakes™
- ☐ Rice Bubbles™
- ☐ Coco Pops™
- ☐ Puffed Wheat

Cereals

- ☐ Special K™
- ☐ Porridge
- ☐ Muesli
- ☐ All-Bran™
- ☐ Frosties™
- ☐ Guardian™
- ☐ Soytana
- ☐ Healthwise for Heart Health

Biscuits

- ☐ Sao™
- ☐ Water crackers
- ☐ Cruskits™
- ☐ Rice cakes
- ☐ Morning Coffee™
- ☐ Milk Arrowroot
- ☐ Shortbread

Biscuits

- ☐ Vita-weat™
- ☐ Rich Tea™
- ☐ Snack Right Fruit Slice
- ☐ Highland Oatmeal

Snacks

- ☐ Dates
- ☐ Glucose
- ☐ Lollies
- ☐ Pretzels
- ☐ Twisties, Burger Rings
- ☐ Muesli bar

Snacks

- ☐ Dried apricots
- ☐ Prunes
- ☐ Nuts
- ☐ Yoghurt
- ☐ Fruity-Bix bars
- ☐ Milk
- ☐ Ice-cream

Fruit

- ☐ Watermelon
- ☐ Dates

Fruit

- ☐ Apples
- ☐ Oranges
- ☐ Bananas
- ☐ Grapes
- ☐ Kiwi fruit
- ☐ Peaches, plums, apricots, cherries

3. Now add up the number of ticks in each column of foods. The foods in the left column have a high GI. If most of your ticks are in this column, you are eating a high GI diet. Consider altering some of your choices to include more of the foods from the column on the right.

Is your diet too high in fat?

Use this fat counter to tally up how much fat your diet contains. Circle all the foods that you could eat in a day, look at the serving size listed and multiply the grams of fat up or down to match your serving size. For example, with milk, if you estimate you might consume 2 cups of regular milk in a day, this supplies you with 20 grams of fat.

Food	Fat content (grams)	How much did you eat?
Dairy Foods		
Milk (250 ml) 1 cup		
regular	10	_____
fat-reduced (<1% fat)	1	_____
skim	0	_____
Yoghurt, 200 gram tub		
Regular	6	_____
Low fat	0	_____
Ice-cream, 2 scoops (100 ml/50 grams)		
regular, vanilla	5	_____
reduced fat, vanilla	3	_____

Food	Fat content (grams)	How much did you eat?
Cheese		
regular block cheese, 20 gram slice	7	_____
reduced-fat block cheese, 30 gram slice	5	_____
low fat slices (per slice)	2	_____
cottage, 2 tablespoons	2	_____
ricotta, 2 tablespoons	2	_____
Cream/sour cream, I tablespoon		
regular	7	_____
fat-reduced	5	_____
Fats and oils		
Butter/margarine, I teaspoon	4	_____
Oil, any type, I tablespoon (20 ml)	20	_____
Cooking spray, per spray	I	_____
Mayonnaise, I tablespoon	6	_____
Salad dressing, I tablespoon	5	_____
Meat		
Beef		
steak, I medium (160 grams), fat trimmed	5	_____
minced beef patty (170 grams), cooked, drained	21	_____
sausage, I thick, grilled (80 grams)	13	_____
topside roast, 2 slices, lean only (80 grams)	5	_____
Lamb		
chump chop, grilled/BBQ, 2, fat trimmed	10	_____
leg, roast meat, lean only, 2 slices (60 grams)	6	_____
loin chop, grilled/BBQ, 2, lean only	6	_____

Food	Fat content (grams)	How much did you eat?
Pork		
bacon, 1 rasher, grilled	6	_____
ham, 1 slice, leg, lean	1	_____
butterfly steak, fat trimmed	3	_____
leg, roast meat, 3 slices (80 grams) lean only	6	_____
large chop, fat trimmed	9	_____
Chicken		
breast, skinless, 150 grams	8	_____
drumstick, skinless	8	_____
thigh, skinless	12	_____
½ barbecue chicken (including skin)	17	_____
Fish		
grilled fish, 1 average fillet	3	_____
salmon, 50 grams	5	_____
fish fingers, 4 grilled	10	_____
fish fillets, 2, crumbed, oven baked		
regular	20	_____
light	16	_____
Snack foods		
Chocolate (50 gram bar)	25	_____
Potato crisps (50 gram bag)	15	_____
Corn chips (50 gram bag)	14	_____
Peanuts, ½ cup (70 grams)	36	_____
French fries, regular serve	20	_____
Pizza, 2 slices, medium pizza	18	_____
Pie/sausage roll	17	_____
Total		

How did you rate?

Less than 40 grams	Excellent. 30 to 40 grams of fat per day is an average range recommended for those trying to lose weight.
41–60 grams	Good. A fat intake in this range is recommended for most adult men and women.
61–80 grams	Acceptable. If you are very active, i.e. doing hard physical work (labouring) or athletic training. It is too much if you are trying to lose weight.
More than 80 grams	You're possibly eating too much fat, unless of course you are Superman or Superwoman!

EATING THE LOW GI WAY

Low GI diets are easy to teach and easy to learn. The basic technique is to swap high GI carbohydrates in your diet with low GI foods. This could mean eating muesli at breakfast instead of wheat flakes, low GI bread instead of normal white or wholemeal bread, or a sparkling apple juice in place of soft drink, for example. We've identified some key points that are crucial in putting the GI into practice. Remember:

- *The GI only relates to carbohydrate-rich foods*

The foods we eat contain three main nutrients—protein, carbohydrate and fat. Some foods, such as meat, are high in protein, while bread is high in carbohydrate and butter is high in fat. It is necessary for us to consume a variety of foods (in varying proportions) to provide all three nutrients, but the GI applies only to high carbohydrate foods. It is impossible for us to measure a GI value for foods which contain negligible carbohydrate. These foods include meats, fish, chicken, eggs, cheese, nuts, oils, cream, butter and most vegetables. There are other nutritional aspects which you could consider in choosing these foods. For example, the amount and type of fats they contain.

- *The GI is not intended to be used in isolation*

The GI of a food does not make it good or bad for us. High GI foods like potato and bread still make valuable nutritional contributions to our diet. And low GI foods like pastry that are high in saturated fat are no better for us because of their low GI. The nutritional benefits of different foods are many and varied, and it is advisable for you to base your food choices on the overall nutritional content of a food, particularly considering the saturated fat, salt and fibre in addition to GI.

- *There is no need to eat only low GI foods*

While most of us will benefit from eating carbohydrate with a low GI at each meal, this doesn't mean consuming it at the exclusion of all other carbohydrate. When we eat a combination of low and high GI carbohydrate foods, like baked beans on toast, fruit and sandwiches, lentils and rice, potatoes and corn, the final

GI of the meal is intermediate. The high GI of foods like potato is moderated by including a low GI carbohydrate at the same meal. For example, if your main meal contains potato with a GI of 90, then choose a low GI dessert like low fat yoghurt with a GI of 33. Let's assume that half the carbohydrate comes from the potato and half from the yoghurt. The GI for the meal then becomes $(50\% \times 90) + (50\% \times 33) = 62$.

- *Consider both the GI of the food and the amount of carbohydrate it contains, i.e. the glycemic load*

For a small number of foods, the normal serving size contains so little carbohydrate that the GI of that carbohydrate is unimportant. This is the case for fruits like watermelon (GI of 72) and for vegetables like parsnips (GI of 97) and pumpkin (GI of 75) which provide about 6 grams of carbohydrate per serving. Small amounts of jam (GI of 51) or honey (GI of 64) also have little glycemic impact. You can calculate the glycemic load by multiplying the GI by the amount of carbohydrate per serve and then dividing by 100. We have included the glycemic load of foods in the tables at the end of the book.

High GI food + Low GI food =
Intermediate GI meal

Glycemic load =
(GI x carbohydrate per serve) ÷ 100

As with kilojoules, the GI value is not precise. What GI values give you is a guide to lowering the GI of your day. A simple change can make a big difference. Look at the type of carbohydrate foods you eat and identify those which you eat the most of (these have the greatest glycemic load). Consider the high carbohydrate foods you consume at each meal and replace at least one with a low GI food (e.g. replace potato with sweet potato). This will result in a significant reduction in the overall GI of your diet. Look at the following table for substitution suggestions.

Substituting low GI for high GI foods

High GI Food	Low GI Alternative
Bread, wholemeal or white	Bread containing a lot of 'grainy bits' such as Burgen™, Performax, Holsom's™, multigrain or Ploughmans™ loaves
Processed breakfast cereal	Unrefined cereal such as rolled oats or muesli or a low GI processed cereal like Guardian™ or All Bran™
Plain biscuits and crackers	Biscuits made with dried fruit and whole grains such as oats
Cakes and muffins	Make them with fruit, oats, whole grain
Potato	Substitute with new potatoes, sweet potatoes, sweet corn and use more pasta and legumes
Rice	Try Basmati or Doongara (Mahatma Premium Classic) rice, or pearled barley, or noodles

Making the change

Some people change their diet easily, but for the majority of us, change of any kind is difficult. Changing our diet is seldom just a matter of giving up certain foods. A healthy diet contains a wide variety of foods but we need to eat them in appropriate proportions. If you are considering changes to your diet, keep these four guidelines in mind:

1. Aim to make changes gradually;

2. Attempt the easiest changes first;

3. Break big goals into a number of smaller, more achievable goals;

4. Accept lapses in your habits.

If you feel like you need some extra help, seek some professional assistance from a dietitian.

5 little tips that make a big difference

- Think of carbohydrate foods as the number one priority in your meals.

- Change a staple in your diet, like bread, to a low GI type to make a big difference to the GI of your day.

- Get in touch with your true appetite and use it to guide the amount of food you eat. Low fat, high fibre, low GI foods fill you up best.

- Try to eat at least two low GI meals each day.

- Mix high GI foods with low GI foods in your meals—the combination will give an overall intermediate GI.

TEN STEPS TO A
HEALTHY HEART DIET

1. Eat more wholegrain breads and cereals.

2. Use beans, peas and lentils more often.

3. Eat lots of fruit and vegetables.

4. Include oily fish at least twice a week
   e.g. salmon, sardines.

5. Minimise saturated fats.

6. Reduce your use of salt.

7. Moderate your alcohol intake.

8. Include nuts in your diet regularly.

9. Use low fat dairy products.

10. Allow yourself a treat a day.

1. Eat more wholegrains

Wholegrains represent the earliest form in which humans consumed cereals. Eaten boiled or roughly pounded to a flour, mixed with water and roasted, they were a form of slow-release carbohydrate with a low GI. They were also filling and sustaining. The advent of high speed roller mills in the Industrial Revolution led to the development of the fine, white flour that is used today. Because the outer seed coat has been removed, the starch in today's flour is readily digested and has a high GI.

We can still get the benefit of wholegrains in our diet today with foods like:

- Barley—e.g. pearl barley in soup
- Whole wheat or cracked wheat e.g. bulgur in tabbouleh
- Oats and rolled oats for breakfast
- Wholegrain breads (the ones with chewy grains and seeds)
    e.g. Burgen™ traditional varieties
    Performax™
    Vogel's™ grain breads
    Multi-Grain™ 9-Grain

If you are making your own bread, GI lowering ingredients to add include linseeds, rolled oats, cornmeal, oat bran, barley meal and kibbled wheat.

2. Use more dried peas, beans and lentils

Dried peas, beans and lentils are collectively known as legumes. They are an excellent food, being:

- rich in low GI carbohydrate
- low in fat
- high in fibre
- low cost

Because they are high in protein, legumes are an ideal substitute for meat. Introduce them to your family gradually by incorporating them in meals with meat e.g. as chilli con carne, a filling for tacos or burritos, and then try some of the delicious vegetarian dishes that can be made using legumes. You could also try:

- 3-bean mix with a salad
- a can of kidney beans in a bolognese sauce
- hommous dip or spread
- pea and ham soup
- potato bake with beans and lean bacon

The special benefits of soy

Foods based on soy beans also have a beneficial role in our defence against heart disease. There are two components of soy beans with the potential to reduce coronary heart disease risk: soy protein and anti-oxidant substances called 'isoflavones'.

Soy foods:

- improve our blood fats—lowering the bad (LDL) cholesterol
- increase the good (HDL) cholesterol
- reduce the accumulation of cholesterol in blood vessels by decreasing LDL oxidation and thereby inflammation
- decrease the tendency to form blood clots or thromboses
- have other health promoting effects on blood vessels

Studies suggest that 1–2 servings of soy protein-rich food each day may be sufficient to provide long term health benefit. Just one cup of soy drink constitutes a serve and can be used as a nutritionally balanced replacement for dairy milk providing it is fortified with calcium. Try:

- soy drink on your breakfast cereal
- a soy banana smoothie
- a soy yoghurt for a snack

3. Eat lots of fruit and vegetables

Plant foods are rich sources of naturally occurring chemicals believed to be involved in disease prevention. Increased consumption of fruit and vegetables is associated with a lower incidence of diseases such as cancer, cardiovascular disease and other age-related diseases.

At least 5 serves a day of fruit and vegetables is recommended. These foods are an essential source of vitamin C but also rich in anti-oxidants and fibre.

Get into a fruit and vegetable habit:

- don't sit down to a main meal without some veges in it
- take an apple and a banana to work
- make a habit of eating some fruit at home when you relax in the evening
- order a side salad with your meal
- buy a new vegetable to try each week
- consider fresh, canned, dried and juiced fruit as sources of fruit for your diet
- chop fresh pineapple or melon into large chunks and keep it on hand in the refrigerator
- prepare a fruit platter for the household to share after a meal

4. Include oily fish at least twice a week

Oily fish are the best source of long chain omega-3 fatty acids. These types of fats are scarcely found in other foods and offer valuable benefits in reducing blood clotting and inflammatory reactions. They can help in the prevention and treatment of heart disease, high blood pressure and rheumatoid arthritis. They are also beneficial in infant brain and eye development.

Fresh fish that are highest in omega-3 fats include:

- Swordfish
- Atlantic Salmon
- Gemfish
- Silver Perch
- Blue Mackerel

Canned fish can also provide substantial amounts of omega-3 fat. Good sources are:

- Mackerel
- Salmon
- Sardines

Smoked salmon and oysters are also a rich source.

Aim to include fish in your diet at least twice a week e.g. a main meal of fresh fish NOT cooked in saturated fat, plus at least one sandwich-sized serve of, say, canned salmon.

5. Reduce saturated fats

Approximately 40 per cent of fats in the Australian diet are saturated fats. This type of fat is believed to be a major cause of high cholesterol levels in our population. The main sources are:

- full cream dairy foods, especially milk, cheese, cream
- ice-cream products
- meat, especially processed meats like sausage, salami
- fat spreads, especially butter, cream cheese and cheese spreads
- take-away foods like deep fried foods, chips, pizza
- snack foods like potato crisps, biscuits, cakes

Make every effort to reduce your intake of saturated fats by eating less of the foods listed previously. Substitute with unsaturated fats where possible, for example:

Instead of:	Substitute:
Butter	monosaturated spread e.g. canola
Dripping/lard	poly- or mono-unsaturated oil
Regular milk	low fat or skim milk
Fatty meat	smaller amounts of leaner cuts e.g. Master Trim Beef or Trim Lamb or New Fashioned Pork
Regular ice-cream	one of the many low fat varieties on the market
Regular cheese	eat it occasionally. Try low fat and reduced fat alternatives

What Fat is That?

The fat in our food is a combination of different types of fatty acids. Depending on which fatty acids predominate, we identify the fat as either saturated, monounsaturated or polyunsaturated.

Saturated	Monounsaturated	Polyunsaturated
Butter	Canola margarine	Polyunsaturated
	Olive margarine	margarines
Solid cooking fats	Canola oil	Sunflower oil
	Olive oil	Safflower oil
Palm oil	Peanut oil	Soybean oil
Coconut oil	Avocado	Walnuts
	Peanuts	Hazelnuts
Copha	Almonds	Brazil nuts
Cocoa butter	Peanut butter	Sunflower seeds

6. Minimise use of salt

It has been estimated that 75 per cent of the salt we eat is not from that which we voluntarily add, but from salt already existing in foods. Bread and butter/margarine, for example, contribute much of the salt we eat. Low salt breads take some time to adjust your tastebuds to, but low salt margarines are easy to find on the supermarket shelves and are not noticeably different in taste.

Foods that are high in salt include:

• canned, bottled and packet soups, sauces and meal and gravy bases, stock cubes
• ham, bacon, sausages and other delicatessen meats
• pizza, meat pies, sausage rolls, fried chicken and other take-away foods
• pickles, chutneys, olives
• snack foods like potato crisps

7. Consume alcohol in moderation

There is no doubt that large quantities of alcohol should be avoided, but several studies have suggested that a moderate alcohol intake exerts a protective effect against heart disease.

People who drink 1–2 standard drinks per day, but not necessarily every day, show a reduced risk of heart disease, with the effect being greatest amongst those with other risk factors for heart disease. The effect of alcohol may be mediated through an increase in the level of 'good' HDL cholesterol. Anti-oxidant substances in red wine which reduce the oxidation of 'bad' LDL cholesterol are also thought to be involved.

It is important to note the finding that 3 or more drinks per day actually increases the risk of death!

A standard drink contains about 10 g of alcohol—the amount found in a 285 ml middy of beer or ⅓ of a bottle of wine, or a 30 ml nip of spirits.

8. Include nuts in your diet

Nuts are a food that many people enjoy but few people eat regularly—a situation that needs to change! Large prospective studies in recent years have found a strong link between higher consumption of nuts and reduced risk of heart disease. Nuts contain a very favourable mix of fatty acids which have a positive effect on blood fat levels.

Nuts are also a good source of other nutrients thought to protect against heart disease including vitamin E, folate, copper and magnesium.

Because they are so nutrient and energy dense, nuts need only be used in small quantities.

While sitting down to a bowl of nuts may not be such a good idea if you are trying to lose weight, consuming small amounts of nuts regularly is quite healthy. Try:

- chopped almonds or pecans in a muesli
- a snack of nuts and dried fruit
- toasted cashews to finish a stir-fry
- a handful of pine nuts scattered over a salad

9. Use low fat dairy products

Dairy foods supply about 70 per cent of our calcium needs and contribute low GI carbohydrate to our diet. Low fat flavoured milks, custards, yoghurts, ice-creams and mousse make great-tasting snacks and desserts.

Men and pre-menopausal women should aim to consume 1000 mg of calcium each day. After meno-pause, optimal intakes for women are up to 1500 mg a day. This requires at least three 1 cup serves of low fat milk product daily.

Low fat milk supplies as much (and usually more) calcium than full cream milk so is entirely suitable for those wanting to increase their calcium intake.

- 1 cup of low fat milk contains 415 mg of calcium and only 0.5 g of fat.
- 1 cup of regular milk contains 295 mg of calcium and 9.7 g of fat.

Full cream milk is recommended for children under 5 years of age because young children have a greater reliance on the kilojoules provided by fat.

10. Allow yourself a treat

Food is meant to be enjoyed!

Allow yourself to indulge in a little of whatever takes your fancy but check with yourself that it is what you really feel like. Indulgences are meant to be enjoyed:

- your favourite cheese and crackers
- a meat pie at the football
- bacon and egg on Sundays
- take-away on Friday night
- a slice of cake at a celebration
- chocolate biscuits with a friend

> The message for heart disease prevention is low fat (low saturated fat), high carbohydrate, high fibre and low GI most of the time!

YOUR LOW GI
STOCKLIST

Nothing affects our day-to-day food choices as much as what we have in the cupboard. Use these ideas as the basis of your shopping list.

Breads

All types of bread are suitable but the lowest GI choices are:

    Original, heavy Burgen™ varieties (Tip Top Bakeries)
    Performax™ Wholemeal loaf (Country Life Bakeries)
    Multigrain™ 9-Grain (Tip Top Bakeries)
    Holsom's™ Wholemeal with Wheatgerm (Tip Top Bakeries)
    Ploughman's™ Whole-Grain (Quality Bakers)

Spreads

If you wish to use a fat spread on your bread choose a margarine labelled 'polyunsaturated' or 'monounsaturated' (and preferably salt reduced).

Breakfast cereals

All-Bran™——try all varieties (Kellogg's)

Guardian™ (Kellogg's)

Special K™ (Kellogg's)

Natural muesli or low fat toasted muesli, e.g. Komplete™ oven baked muesli (Kellogg's)

Rolled oats and oat bran

Cereals enriched with psyllium, when eaten as part of a low fat diet, lower levels of bad cholesterol but maintain good cholesterol levels.

Fruits

Lowest GI fresh fruit choices include:

Apples	Plums	Grapefruit
Cherries	Peaches	Kiwifruit
Pears	Oranges	Grapes

Dried fruits——sultanas, dried apricots, fruit medley, raisins, prunes etc.

Canned peaches, pears, apples are a useful standby.

Fruit juices are also suitable but shouldn't be drunk to excess —generally only 1–2 cups per day.

Rice & grains

Basmati or Doongara rice

Pasta——fresh and dried

Noodles

Pearl barley

Legumes

Dried lentils, chick peas, cannellini beans

A variety of canned legumes (kidney beans, mixed beans, baked beans)

Vegetables

All vegetables are good for you—fresh, frozen and canned. Raw salad vegetables are available partially prepared to make a quick addition to the meal. Canned vegetables—tomatoes, asparagus, peas, corn, beetroot, mushrooms and crisp, canned mixed veges are always handy to boost the vegetable content of a meal. Other convenient vegetable products are:

    tomato paste

    tomato purée and bottled tomato pasta sauces

    frozen vegetables

Meats

Any meat trimmed of all visible fat

Low fat minced meat

Skinless chicken or turkey

Lean bacon

Lean cold meats—ham, corned beef, pastrami, turkey or chicken breast

Fish

All fresh fish is recommended

Canned fish such as salmon, mackerel, tuna, herrings, sardines

Smoked fish, like smoked cod

Frozen fish products that have used poly- or monounsaturated oils in their preparation (check labels carefully!)

Seafood

Most seafood is suitable to include regularly but avoid if battered or crumbed or in a creamy sauce.

Calamari and octopus are recommended only once per week if you have high cholesterol.

Dairy foods

Milk—fat-reduced and skim

Yoghurt—low fat, fruit and natural

UHT skim milk or skim milk powder—easy to use in cooking

Canned evaporated skim milk

Low fat ice cream

Cottage cheese, low fat ricotta

Low fat block and processed cheese (check the label for those which are less than 10 per cent fat.)

Flavourings, sauces & dressings

Spices—curry powder, cumin, turmeric, mustard etc.

Herbs—oregano, basil, thyme etc.

Bottled minced ginger, chilli and garlic

Sauces e.g. Worcestershire, soy, chilli, oyster, BBQ, hoisin

Stock base (ready-prepared tetra brick pack) or powders

Low oil salad dressings

A WEEK OF LOW GI EATING

This week of menus shows you how to achieve a healthy heart diet with a low GI. You can use the menus for ideas for your own meal choices or follow them closely to try out the low GI diet.

We have included between-meal snacks in most of the menus as they can be part of a normal healthy diet.

Each menu is designed to be:

- **low in fat, especially saturated fat**
  We've kept the total amount of fat down to provide less than 30 per cent of total kilojoules, according to current recommendations. Saturated fat content is less than 20 grams per day.

- **low in kilojoules**

  These menus provide a total daily kilojoule intake of between 5800–7000 kJ (1400–1700 cal) which is a minimum amount for most people. Be guided by your appetite to adjust quantities to suit yourself.

- **high in carbohydrate with a low GI**

  The carbohydrate content of these menus provides at least 50 per cent of total kilojoule intake. This means an intake of at least 200 grams of carbohydrate each day. The emphasis is on low GI carbohydrate choices.

Generally, beverages are included only where they make a significant nutrient or kilojoule contribution. Supplement the menus with a range of fluids such as water, tea, coffee, herbal tea, cereal coffee, mineral water and soda with lemon or lime juice.

Recipe ideas for dishes marked with an asterisk are given on pages 92–94.

Monday Menu

Total Energy:	6300 kJ
Saturated Fat:	10 g
Carbohydrate:	230 g
Fibre:	44 g

Breakfast: A bowl of Guardian™ with a sliced banana and low fat milk
Slice of grain toast with unsaturated margarine

Morning snack   A couple of oatmeal cookies

Lunch: Two slices of fresh grain bread filled with tuna, lettuce and canola mayonnaise. Team with a snack pack of canned fruit

Dinner: A large bowl of steaming, thick minestrone soup served with crusty Italian bread and a salad with vinaigrette dressing

Night snack   One scoop of low fat, low GI ice-cream with fresh fruit salad

Tuesday Menu

Total Energy:	6400 kJ
Saturated Fat:	10 g
Carbohydrate:	230 g
Fibre:	33 g

Breakfast: Top a couple of slices of Burgen™ fruit loaf with low fat ricotta cheese and a finely sliced pear. Finish with a hot chocolate made with low fat milk

Lunch: A baked bean jaffle (spray the jaffle maker with cooking spray) and a cup of fresh pineapple chunks

Afternoon snack A low fat apple muffin

Dinner: Barbecued Beef Kebabs* with Quick Rice Combo*

Night snack Lemon sorbet

* See recipe on pages 93–94

Wednesday Menu

Total Energy:	6000 kJ
Saturated Fat:	12 g
Carbohydrate:	200 g
Fibre:	30 g

Breakfast: A bowl of porridge with a tablespoon of sultanas and low fat milk. Team it with a glass of orange juice

Lunch: Two slices of grain bread spread with avocado, topped with beetroot, grated carrot and lettuce. A piece of fresh fruit and water

Afternoon snack A tub of low fat yoghurt

Dinner: Quick Vegetarian Pizza*

Night snack A small handful (30 g) of almonds and a glass of sparkling apple juice

* See recipe on page 92

Thursday Menu

Total Energy:	7000 kJ
Saturated Fat:	12 g
Carbohydrate:	230 g
Fibre:	40 g

Breakfast: Toast 2 slices of grain bread and top with a smear of avocado, sliced tomato and black pepper. Add a piece of fresh fruit and a drink

Lunch: Try a bowl of lentil and vegetable soup with Lebanese flat bread

Afternoon snack   An orange

Dinner: Salmon Cakes* served with a medley of baby corn, snow peas, sliced carrots and shallots. Drizzle with sweet chilli sauce if desired

Night snack   Low fat ice cream in a cone

* See recipe on page 93

Friday Menu

Total Energy:	5800 kJ
Saturated Fat:	15 g
Carbohydrate:	180 g
Fibre:	32 g

Breakfast: Top a couple of slices of grain toast with baked beans and a poached egg. Add a small glass of grapefruit juice or fresh grapefruit

Lunch: Two slices of sourdough rye bread, smear of light cream cheese, sliced smoked salmon and a side salad

Afternoon snack A slice of raisin toast with a scrape of margarine

Dinner: Easy Creamy Pasta* with tomato topping and side salad

Night snack A tub of frozen yoghurt

* See recipe on page 92

Saturday Menu

Total Energy:	7000 kJ
Saturated Fat:	8 g
Carbohydrate:	230 g
Fibre:	44 g

Breakfast: A bowl of Healthwise for the Heart™ with low fat milk, low fat berry yoghurt and a handful of strawberries

Lunch: A Lebanese roll filled with felafel, hommous, tomato, lettuce, tabbouleh and chilli sauce

Afternoon snack Small bunch of grapes

Dinner: Moroccan Lamb and Spicy Rice* and steamed vegetables

Night snack 2 fresh plums

* See recipes on page 93

Sunday Menu

Total Energy:	6600 kJ
Saturated Fat:	12 g
Carbohydrate:	175 g
Fibre:	30 g

Breakfast: A bowl of fresh fruit salad topped with 100 g low fat fruit yoghurt. Add a reduced fat apple and sultana muffin.

Lunch: Whip up an omelette and team it with a couple of slices of grain bread. Combine 1 whole egg with 2 beaten egg whites. Cook lightly in an omelette pan and top with diced tomato, shallots and a sprinkle of grated reduced fat cheese. Finish under the grill

Afternoon snack A banana

Dinner: Pan-cook or barbecue a fish cutlet drizzled with a little olive oil, lemon juice, salt and pepper. Serve with canned new potatoes and steamed seasonal vegetables

Night snack A glass of fruit juice and a small scoop of cashews

QUICK MEAL IDEAS

These recipe ideas are used in the previous menu plans. The quantities are only a rough guide and can be adjusted to taste.

Easy Creamy Pasta

Put 250 g of broad fettuccine noodles on to boil. Combine ¼ cup of fresh ricotta, ¼ cup of low fat natural yoghurt, ¼ cup of grated parmesan and 3 tspns of margarine. Stir this mixture through the drained pasta, adding some sautéed onion and garlic for extra flavour if desired. A quick topping idea is bottled pasta sauce.

Serves 4.

Quick Vegetarian Pizza

Sauté a diced onion, a clove of crushed garlic and strips of green capsicum. Add 4 thinly sliced mushrooms and basil and oregano to taste and cook 5 minutes. Stir in a small can of red kidney beans.

Sprinkle a pizza base with ½ cup of grated reduced fat mozzarella or pizza cheese. Spoon the bean mixture over. Pour over about ½ cup of bottled tomato puree and top with another ½ cup of cheese. Bake 10–15 minutes in a hot oven.

Serves 4.

Salmon Cakes

Combine a 200 g can of salmon with half a finely diced onion, ½ cup of mashed potato, 2 tspns chopped parsley and 1 egg. Shape into patties and cook in a pan sprayed with cooking spray.

Serves 2.

Moroccan Lamb & Spicy Rice

Coat about 120 g of trim lamb (e.g. lamb fillet) with a commercial Moroccan spice blend and pan-fry in a little oil. Remove to a plate and keep warm. In the same pan, sauté a finely sliced onion until golden, collecting the spice remaining in the pan. Add 1 cup of cooked Basmati rice and ½ cup of cooked baby peas. Stir over heat to combine and heat through. Serve topped with the lamb cut into strips and freshly steamed vegetables.

Serves 1.

Quick Rice Combo

Stir fry 2 rashers of trimmed, diced bacon, 1 small red capsicum, diced, 2 chopped shallots, 1 cup of frozen corn/peas and 1 cup of bean sprouts. Add 2 cups of cooked Doongara rice, drizzle with soy sauce and serve.

Serves 2.

Barbecued Beef Kebabs

Marinate approximately 500 g of diced beef (e.g. rump, fillet) in ½ cup red wine, 1 tbspn vinegar, 1 tbspn olive oil, 1 tspn Worcestershire sauce, 2 tbspns tomato sauce, crushed garlic and black pepper. Thread onto skewers alternately with button mushrooms, diced capsicum and diced onion. Grill or barbecue and serve with Quick Rice Combo.

Serves 4.

LET'S TALK GLYCEMIC LOAD

When we eat a meal containing carbohydrate, our blood glucose rises and falls. The extent to which it rises and remains high is critically important to health and depends on two things: the *amount* of a carbohydrate in the meal and the *nature* (GI) of that carbohydrate. Both are equally important determinants of changes in blood glucose levels.

Researchers at Harvard University have come up with a way of combining and describing these two factors with the term 'glycemic load'. Glycemic load is the product of the GI and carbohydrate per serve of food. You'll find it listed in the tables at the back of this book.

Glycemic load is calculated simply by multiplying the GI of a food by the amount of carbohydrate per serving and dividing by 100.

Glycemic load = (GI × carbohydrate per serving) ÷ 100

For example, an apple has a GI of 40 and contains 15 grams of carbohydrate per serve. Its glycemic load is (40 × 15) ÷ 100 = 6. A potato has a GI of 90 and 20 grams of carbohydrate per serve. It has a glycemic load of (90 × 20) ÷ 100 = 18.

The glycemic load is greatest for those foods which provide the most carbohydrate, particularly those we tend to eat in large quantities. Compare the glycemic load of the following foods to see how the serving size as well as the GI are significant in determining the glycemic response:

Rice—1 cup of boiled Calrose rice (150 g) contains 43 g carbohydrate and has a GI of 83. The glycemic load is (83 × 43) ÷ 100 = 36.

Spaghetti—1 serve (150 g) of cooked spaghetti contains 48 g carbohydrate and has a GI of 44. The glycemic load is (44 × 48) ÷ 100 = 21.

Some nutritionists have argued that the glycemic load is an improvement on the GI because it provides an estimate of both quantity and quality of carbohydrate (the GI gives us just quality) in a diet. In large scale studies from Harvard University, however, the risk of disease was predicted by both the GI of the overall diet as well as the glycemic load. The use of the glycemic load strengthened the relationship, suggesting that the more frequent the consumption of high carbohydrate, high GI foods, the more adverse the health outcome.

Don't make the mistake of using GL alone. If you do, you might find yourself eating a diet with very little carbohydrate but a lot of fat, especially saturated fat, and excessive amounts of protein. Use the glycemic index to compare foods of similar nature (e.g. bread with bread) and use the glycemic load when you note a high GI but low carbohydrate content per serve (e.g. pumpkin).

THE GI & GL TABLES

These tables are an A to Z listing of the GI and GL of foods commonly eaten in Australia and New Zealand. Approximately 400 different foods are listed.

The GI value shown next to each food is the average for that food using glucose as the standard, i.e., glucose has a GI value of 100, with other foods rated accordingly. The average may represent the mean of ten studies of that food worldwide or only two to four studies. In a few instances, Australian data are different from the rest of the world and we show our data rather than the average. Rice and porridge fall into this category.

The glycemic load (GL = carbohydrate content × GI ÷ 100) shows you the blood glucose response to a serving of a food. The higher the glycemic load the higher your blood glucose level will rise. This is calculated using a 'nominal' serving size and the carbohydrate content of that serve, both of which are also listed in the tables. In this way, you can choose foods with either a low GI and/or a low GL.

We've also included foods that contain very little carbohydrate and have therefore been automatically omitted from previous editions. However, so many people ask us for the GI of these foods, we decided to include them and show their GI as 0, indicated by a zero [0]. Many vegetables such as avocados and broccoli and protein foods such as chicken, cheese and tuna are among the low or no carbohydrate category.

If you can't find a GI value for a food you eat regularly, please write to the manufacturer and encourage them to have the GI of the food tested by an accredited laboratory such as Sydney University Glycemic Index Research Service (SUGiRS) (www.glycemicindex.com).

You might also encourage companies to join the GI symbol program (www.gisymbol.com.au), which flags healthy foods that have been properly tested.

The GI values in these tables are correct at the time of publication. However, the formulation of commercial foods can change and the GI may be altered. You can rely on those foods showing the GI symbol. You will find revised and new data on our website (www. glycemicindex.com).

FOOD	GI	NOMINAL SERVE SIZE	AVAILABLE CARB PER SERVE	GL PER SERVE
All-Bran™, breakfast cereal	30	30 g	15	4
All-Bran Fruit 'n' Oats™, breakfast cereal	39	30 g	17	7
All-Bran Soy 'n' Fibre™, breakfast cereal	33	30 g	14	4
Angel food cake, 1 slice	67	50 g	29	19
Apple, raw, 1 medium	38*	120 g	15	6
Apple, dried	29	60 g	34	10
Apple juice, pure, unsweetened	40	250 ml	28	11
Apple muffin	44	60 g	29	13
Apple, oat and sultana muffin (from packet mix)	54	50 g	26	14
Apricots, raw, 3 medium	57	168 g	13	7
Apricots, canned in light syrup	64	120 g	19	12
Apricots, dried	30	60 g	27	8
Apricot, coconut and honey muffin (from mix)	60	50 g	26	16
Arborio, risotto rice, white, boiled	69	150 g	43	29
Bagel, white	72	70 g	35	25
Baked beans, canned in tomato sauce	48*	150 g	17	8
Banana, raw, 1 large	52*	120 g	26	13
Banana cake, 1 slice	47	80 g	38	18
Banana, oat and honey muffin (from packet mix)	65	50 g	26	17
Barley, pearled, boiled	25*	150 g	32	8
Basmati rice, white, boiled, 1 cup	58	150 g	42	24
Beef	[0]	120 g	0	0
Beer	[0]	150 ml	0	0

* Average

FOOD	GI	NOMINAL SERVE SIZE	AVAILABLE CARB PER SERVE	GL PER SERVE
Beetroot, canned	64	80 g	7	5
Bengal gram dhal, chickpea	11	150 g	36	4
Black bean soup	64	250 ml	27	17
Black beans, boiled	30	150 g	25	5
Blackbread (Riga)	76	30 g	13	10
Blackeyed beans, soaked, boiled	42	150 g	29	12
Blueberry muffin	59	57 g	29	17
Bran Flakes™, breakfast cereal	74	30 g	18	13
Bran muffin	60	57 g	24	15
Breton™ wheat crackers	67	25 g	14	10
Broad beans	79	80 g	11	9
Broken rice, white, cooked in rice cooker	86	150 g	43	37
Buckwheat, boiled	54*	150 g	30	16
Buckwheat, pancakes, gluten-free, made from packet mix	102	77 g	22	22
Bulghur, boiled 20 min	48*	150 g	26	12
Bun, hamburger	61	30 g	15	9
Bürgen® Oat Bran & Honey	49	40 g	13	7
Bürgen® Soy-Lin, kibbled soy (8%) and linseed (8%) loaf	36	30 g	9	3
Bürgen® Fruit Loaf	44	30 g	13	6
Bürgen® Mixed Grain	49*	30 g	11	6
Burger Rings™, barbeque-flavoured	90	50 g	31	28
Butter beans, dried, boiled	31*	150 g	20	6
Calrose rice, white, medium grain, boiled	83	150 g	42	35
Capellini pasta, boiled	45	180 g	45	20

* Average

FOOD	GI	NOMINAL SERVE SIZE	AVAILABLE CARB PER SERVE	GL PER SERVE
Capsicum	[0]	80 g	0	0
Carrots, peeled, boiled	41*	80 g	5	2
Cheese	[0]	120 g	0	0
Cherries, raw	63	60 g	6	4
Chickpeas, canned in brine	42	150 g	22	9
Chickpeas, dried, boiled	28*	150 g	24	7
Chicken nuggets, frozen, reheated in microwave oven 5 min	46	100 g	16	7
Chocolate, plain, milk	43*	50 g	28	12
Chocolate, white, Milky Bar®	44	50 g	29	13
Chocolate butterscotch muffins, made from packet mix	53	50 g	28	15
Chocolate cake made from packet mix with chocolate frosting	38	111 g	52	20
Chocolate mousse, 2% fat	31	50 g	11	3
Chocolate pudding, instant made from packet with whole milk	47	100 g	16	7
Coca Cola®, soft drink	53	250 ml	26	14
Coco Pops™	77	30 g	26	20
Condensed milk, sweetened, full-fat	61	50 ml	28	17
Cordial, orange, reconstituted	66	250 ml	20	13
Corn chips, plain, salted	42	50 g	25	11
Cornflakes™, breakfast cereal	77	30 g	25	20
Cornflakes Crunchy Nut™, breakfast cereal	72	30 g	24	17
Cornmeal, boiled in salted water 2 min	68	150 g	13	9
Corn pasta, gluten-free, boiled	78	180 g	42	32
Corn Pops™, breakfast cereal	80	30 g	26	21

* Average

FOOD	GI	NOMINAL SERVE SIZE	AVAILABLE CARB PER SERVE	GL PER SERVE
Corn Thins, puffed corn cakes, gluten-free	87	25 g	20	18
Couscous, boiled 5 min	65*	150 g	33	21
Cranberry juice cocktail	52	250 ml	31	16
Crispix™, breakfast cereal	87	30 g	25	22
Croissant	67	57 g	26	17
Crumpet, white	69	50 g	19	13
Crunchy Nut Cornflakes™ bar	72	30 g	26	19
Crunchy Nut™ Cornflakes	72	30 g	24	17
Cupcake, strawberry-iced	73	38 g	26	19
Custard, home made from milk, (wheat starch), and sugar	43	100 ml	17	7
Custard, prepared from powder with whole milk, No Bake™ (Nestlé)	35	100 ml	17	6
Custard, TRIM™, reduced-fat	37	100 ml	15	6
Custard apple, raw, flesh only	54	120 g	19	10
Dark rye, Blackbread (Riga)	76	30 g	13	10
Dark rye, Schinkenbrot (Riga)	86	30 g	14	12
Dates, dried	103	60 g	40	42
Desiree potato, peeled, boiled 35 min	101	150 g	17	17
Dietworks™ Hazelnut & Apricot bar	42	50 g	22	9
Digestives plain, 2 biscuits	59*	25 g	16	10
Doongara, rice, white, boiled	56*	150 g	42	24
Egg Custard, prepared from powdered mix with whole milk, no bake	35	100 ml	17	6
Eggs	[0]	120 g	0	0
Ensure™, vanilla drink	48	250 ml	34	16

* Average

FOOD	GI	NOMINAL SERVE SIZE	AVAILABLE CARB PER SERVE	GL PER SERVE
Ensure™ bar, chocolate fudge brownie	43	38 g	20	8
Ensure Plus™, vanilla drink	40	237 ml	40	19
Ensure Pudding™, old-fashioned vanilla	36	113 g	26	9
Fanta®, orange soft drink	68	250 ml	34	23
Fettuccine, egg, cooked	32	180 g	46	15
Figs, dried, tenderised	61	60 g	26	16
Fish	[0]	120 g	0	0
Fish fillet, crumbed (Maggi)	43	85 g	16	7
Fish Fingers	38	100 g	19	7
French baguette, white, plain	95	30 g	15	15
French fries, frozen, reheated in microwave	75	150 g	29	22
French vanilla ice-cream, premium, 16% fat (Sara Lee)	38	50 g	9	3
Froot Loops™, breakfast cereal	69	30 g	26	18
Fruche, diet, vanilla	31	200 g	12	4
Frosties™, sugar-coated Cornflakes	55	30 g	26	15
Fruit bites, apple and sultana, Arnott's	45	35 g	25	11
Fructose, pure	19*	10 g	10	2
Vanilla cake made from packet mix with vanilla frosting	42	111 g	58	24
Fruit cocktail, canned (Canada)	55	120 g	16	9
Fruit Fingers, Heinz Kidz™, banana	61	30 g	20	12
Fruit loaf, Bürgen™	44	30 g	13	6
Fruit Loaf, dense continental style wheat bread with dried fruit	47	30 g	15	7
Fruit and Spice Loaf, thick sliced	54	30 g	15	8

* Average

FOOD	GI	NOMINAL SERVE SIZE	AVAILABLE CARB PER SERVE	GL PER SERVE
Gatorade® sports drink	78	250 ml	15	12
Glucodin™ glucose tablets	102	10 g	10	10
Gluten-free white bread, sliced	80	30 g	15	12
Gluten-free multigrain bread	79	30 g	13	10
Gluten-free muesli, with 1.5% fat milk	39	30 g	19	7
Gluten-free corn pasta	78	180 g	42	32
Gluten-free rice and maize pasta	76	180 g	49	37
Gluten-free split pea and soy pasta shells	29	180 g	31	9
Gluten-free spaghetti, rice and split pea, canned in tomato sauce	68	220 g	27	19
Glutinous rice, white, cooked in rice cooker	98	150 g	32	31
Gnocchi, cooked (Latina)	68	180 g	48	33
Golden Wheats™, breakfast cereal	71	30 g	23	16
Grapefruit, raw	25	120 g	11	3
Grapefruit juice, unsweetened	48	250 ml	20	9
Grapes, green	46*	120 g	18	8
Green pea soup, canned	66	250 ml	41	27
Guardian™, breakfast cereal	37	30 g	12	5
Hamburger bun	61	30 g	15	9
Haricot/navy beans, cooked/canned	38*	150 g	31	12
Healthwise™ breakfast cereal for bowel health	66	30 g	18	12
Healthwise™ breakfast cereal for heart health	48	30 g	19	9
Helga's™ Classic Seed Loaf	68	30 g	14	9
Helga's™ traditional wholemeal bread	70	30 g	13	9

* Average

FOOD	GI	NOMINAL SERVE SIZE	AVAILABLE CARB PER SERVE	GL PER SERVE
Honey, Yellow Box honey	35	25 g	18	6
Honey, Stringybark	44	25 g	21	9
Honey, Ironbark	48	25 g	15	7
Honey, Capilano	64*	25 g	17	11
Honey & Oat bread, Vogel's	55	30 g	14	7
Honey Rice Bubbles™, breakfast cereal	77	30 g	27	20
Honey Smacks™, breakfast cereal	71	30 g	23	11
Ice-cream, Norco Prestige Light rich Vanilla	47	50 g	10	5
Ice-cream, Norco Prestige Light Toffee	37	50 g	14	5
Ice-cream, Norco Prestige Macadamia	39	50 g	12	5
Ice-cream, regular, average	61*	50 g	13	8
Ice-cream, Peter's light and creamy	44	100 ml	14	6
Ice-cream, premium, French vanilla, 16% fat	38	50 g	9	3
Ice-cream, premium, 'ultra chocolate', 15% fat	37	50 g	9	4
Instant mashed potato, prepared	69*	150 g	20	17
Instant rice, white, cooked 6 min	87	150 g	42	29
Ironman PR bar®, chocolate	39	65 g	26	10
Isostar® sports drink	70	250 ml	18	13
Jam, apricot fruit spread, reduced sugar	55	30 g	13	7
Jam, strawberry, regular	51	30 g	20	10
Jasmine rice, white, long-grain, cooked in rice cooker	109	150 g	42	46
Jatz™, plain salted cracker biscuits	55	25 g	17	10

* Average

FOOD	GI	NOMINAL SERVE SIZE	AVAILABLE CARB PER SERVE	GL PER SERVE
Jelly Beans	78*	30 g	28	22
Jevity™, fibre-enriched drink	48	237 ml	36	17
Just Right™, breakfast cereal	60	30 g	22	13
Just Right Just Grains™, breakfast cereal	62	30 g	23	14
Kaiser rolls	73	30 g	16	12
Kavli™ Norwegian Crispbread	71	25 g	16	12
Kidney beans, canned	52	150 g	17	9
Kidz™, Heinz, Fruit Fingers, banana	61	30 g	20	12
Kidney beans, boiled	28*	150 g	25	7
Kiwi fruit, raw	58	120 g	12	7
Komplete™, breakfast cereal	48	30 g	21	10
K-Time Just Right™ breakfast cereal bar	72	30 g	24	17
K-Time Strawberry Crunch™ breakfast cereal bar	77	30 g	25	19
Lactose, pure	46*	10 g	10	5
Lamb	[0]	120 g	0	0
Lamingtons, sponge dipped in chocolate and coconut	87	50 g	29	25
L.E.A.N Fibergy™ bar, Harvest Oat	45	50 g	29	13
L.E.A.N Life long Nutribar™, Peanut Crunch	30	40 g	19	6
L.E.A.N Life long Nutribar™, Chocolate Crunch	32	40 g	19	6
L.E.A.N Nutrimeal™, drink powder, Dutch Chocolate	26	250 g	13	3
Lebanese bread, white, 1 round	75	83 g	45	34
Lentils, canned, green	52	50 g	17	9

* Average

THE NEW GLUCOSE REVOLUTION TABLES

FOOD	GI	NOMINAL SERVE SIZE	AVAILABLE CARB PER SERVE	GL PER SERVE
Lentils, green, dried, boiled	30*	150 g	17	5
Lentils, boiled	29*	150 g	18	5
Lentils, red, boiled	26	150 g	18	5
Life Savers®, peppermint	70	30 g	30	21
Light rye bread	68	30 g	14	10
Lima beans, baby, frozen, reheated in microwave oven	32	150 g	30	10
Linguine pasta, thick, cooked	46*	180 g	48	22
Linguine pasta, thin, cooked	52*	180 g	45	23
Lowan honey-toasted breakfast cereal	68	50 g	37	25
Lucozade®, original, sparkling glucose drink	95	250 ml	42	40
Lungkow beanthread noodles	26	180 g	45	12
Lychees, canned in syrup, drained	79	120 g	20	16
M & M's®, peanut	33	30 g	17	6
Macaroni, plain, boiled	47*	180 g	48	23
Macaroni and Cheese, made from mix	64	180 g	51	32
Maltose, 50 g	105	10 g	10	11
Mango raw	51*	120 g	17	8
Maple syrup, Pure Canadian	54	24 g	18	10
Marmalade, orange	48	30 g	20	9
Mars Bar®	62	60 g	40	25
Melba toast	70	30 g	23	16
Milk, full-fat cow's milk, fresh	31	250 ml	12	4
Milk, skim	32	250 ml	13	4
Milk, low fat, chocolate, with sugar, Lite White™	34	250 ml	26	9
Milk, condensed, sweetened	61	50 ml	28	17

* Average

FOOD	GI	NOMINAL SERVE SIZE	AVAILABLE CARB PER SERVE	GL PER SERVE
Milk Arrowroot™ biscuits	69	25 g	18	12
Milky Bar®, plain, white chocolate	44	50 g	29	13
Millet, boiled	71	150 g	36	25
Milo™, chocolate powder, dissolved in water	54	250 ml	16	9
Milo™, ready to drink bottle	30	600 ml	66	20
Mini Wheats™, whole wheat breakfast cereal	58	30 g	21	12
Mini Wheats™, blackcurrant whole wheat breakfast cereal	72	30 g	21	15
Mixed grain loaf, Bürgen®	49*	30 g	11	6
Morning Coffee™, 3 biscuits	79	25 g	19	15
Mousse, butterscotch, reduced fat	36	50 g	10	4
Mousse, chocolate, reduced fat	31	50 g	11	3
Mousse, hazelnut, reduced fat	36	50 g	10	4
Mousse, mango, reduced fat	33	50 g	11	4
Mousse, mixed berry, reduced fat	36	50 g	10	4
Mousse, strawberry, reduced fat	32	50 g	10	3
Muesli bar containing dried fruit	61	30 g	21	13
Muesli, gluten-free with 1.5% fat milk	39	30 g	19	7
Muesli, toasted (Purina)	43	30 g	17	7
Muesli, Swiss Formula, natural	56	30 g	16	9
Multi-Grain 9-Grain	43	30 g	14	6
Mung bean noodles (Lungkow beanthread), dried, boiled	39	180 g	45	18
Naytura, natural muesli	65	60 g	33	21
Nesquik™ powder, chocolate dissolved in 1.5% fat milk	41	250 ml	11	5

* Average

FOOD	GI	NOMINAL SERVE SIZE	AVAILABLE CARB PER SERVE	GL PER SERVE
Nesquik™ powder, strawberry dissolved in 1.5% fat milk	35	250 ml	12	4
New potato, unpeeled and boiled 20 min	78	150 g	21	16
New potato, canned, heated in microwave 3 min	65	150 g	18	12
No Bake Egg Custard, prepared from powder with whole milk	35	100 ml	17	6
Noodles, instant 'two-minute' Maggi®	47*	180 g	40	19
Noodles, mung bean (Lungkow beanthread), dried, boiled	39	180 g	45	18
Noodles, rice, freshly made, boiled	40	180 g	39	15
Norco Ice-cream, Prestige Light rich Vanilla	47	50 g	10	5
Norco Ice-cream, Prestige Light Toffee	37	50 g	14	5
Norco Ice-cream, Prestige Macadamia	39	50 g	12	5
Nutella®, chocolate hazelnut spread	33	20 g	12	4
Nutrigrain™, breakfast cereal	66	30 g	15	10
Oat 'n' Honey Bake™, breakfast cereal	77	30 g	17	13
Oat Bran & Honey Loaf bread, Bürgen®	49	40 g	13	7
Oat bran, raw	55*	10 g	5	3
Orange, 1 medium	42*	120 g	11	5
Orange cordial, reconstituted	66	250 ml	20	13
Orange juice, unsweetened, reconstituted	53	250 ml	18	9
Pancakes, prepared from shake mix	67	70 g	23	15

* Average

FOOD	GI	NOMINAL SERVE SIZE	AVAILABLE CARB PER SERVE	GL PER SERVE
Pancakes, buckwheat, gluten-free, made from packet mix	102	77 g	22	22
Parsnips	97	80 g	12	12
Party pies, beef, cooked	45	100 g	27	12
Pastry, plain	59	57 g	26	15
Paw paw, raw	59*	120 g	8	5
Peach, fresh, 1 large	42*	120 g	11	5
Peach, canned in heavy syrup	58	120 g	15	9
Peach, canned in light syrup	52	120 g	18	9
Peach, canned in reduced-sugar syrup, SPC Lite	62	120 g	17	11
Peanuts, roasted, salted	14*	50 g	6	1
Pear, raw	38*	120 g	11	4
Pear halves, canned in natural juice	43	120 g	13	5
Pear halves, canned in reduced-sugar syrup, (SPC Lite)	25	120 g	14	4
Peas, dried, boiled	22	150 g	9	2
Peas, green, frozen, boiled	48*	80 g	7	3
Pecans (raw)	10	50 g	3	1
Pelde brown rice, boiled	76	150 g	38	29
Performax™ bread	38	30 g	13	5
Pikelets, Golden brand	85	40 g	21	18
Pineapple, raw	59*	120 g	10	6
Pineapple juice, unsweetened	46	250 ml	34	15
Pinto beans, canned in brine	45	150 g	22	10
Pinto beans, dried, boiled	39	150 g	26	10
Pita bread, white	57	30 g	17	10
Pizza, cheese	60	100 g	27	16

* Average

FOOD	GI	NOMINAL SERVE SIZE	AVAILABLE CARB PER SERVE	GL PER SERVE
Pizza, Super Supreme, pan (11.4% fat)	36	100 g	24	9
Pizza, Super Supreme, thin and crispy (13.2 % fat)	30	100 g	22	7
Ploughman's™ Wholegrain bread, original recipe	47	30 g	14	7
Ploughman's™ Wholemeal bread, smooth milled	64	30 g	13	9
Plums, raw	39*	120 g	12	5
Pontiac potato, peeled, boiled 35 min	88	150 g	18	16
Pontiac potato, peeled and microwave on high for 6–7.5 min	79	150 g	18	14
Pontiac potato, peeled, cubed, boiled 15 min, mashed	91	150 g	20	18
Pop Tarts™, Double Chocolate	70	50 g	36	25
Popcorn, plain, cooked in microwave oven	72*	20 g	11	8
Pork	[0]	120 g	0	0
Porridge made from whole oats	55	250 g	21	12
Potato crisps, plain, salted	54*	50 g	21	11
Pound cake	54	53 g	28	15
Poweraid®	65	250 ml	20	13
Power Bar®, chocolate	56*	65 g	42	24
Pretzels, oven-baked, traditional wheat flavour	83	30 g	20	16
Prunes, pitted, 6	29	60 g	33	10
Pudding, instant, chocolate, made from powder and whole milk	47	100 g	16	7
Pudding, instant, vanilla, made from powder and whole milk	40	100 g	16	6

* Average

FOOD	GI	NOMINAL SERVE SIZE	AVAILABLE CARB PER SERVE	GL PER SERVE
Pudding, Sustagen™, instant vanilla, made from powdered mix	27	250 g	47	13
Puffed crispbread	81	25 g	19	15
Puffed rice cakes, white	82	25 g	21	17
Puffed Wheat, breakfast cereal	80	30 g	21	17
Pumpernickel rye kernel bread	50*	30 g	12	6
Pumpkin	75	80 g	4	3
Quik™, chocolate (Nestlé, Australia), dissolved in 1.5% fat milk	41	250 ml	11	5
Quik™, strawberry (Nestlé, Australia), dissolved in 1.5% fat milk	35	250 ml	12	4
Raisins	64	60 g	44	28
Ravioli, durum wheat flour, meat filled, boiled	39	180 g	38	15
Real Fruit Bars, strawberry processed fruit bars	90	30 g	26	23
Rice and maize pasta, Ris'O'Mais, gluten-free	76	180 g	49	37
Rice Bran, extruded	19	30 g	14	3
Rice Bubbles™, breakfast cereal	87	30 g	26	22
Rice Bubble Treat™ bar	63	30 g	24	15
Rice cakes, white	82	25 g	21	17
Rice Krispies™, breakfast cereal	82	30 g	26	22
Rice noodles, freshly made, boiled	40	180 g	39	15
Rice pasta, brown, boiled 16 min	92	180 g	38	35
Rice vermicelli, dried, boiled	58	180 g	39	22
Rich Tea, 2 biscuits	55	25 g	19	10
Risotto rice, arborio, boiled	69	150 g	43	29

* Average

FOOD	GI	NOMINAL SERVE SIZE	AVAILABLE CARB PER SERVE	GL PER SERVE
Rockmelon/cantaloupe, raw	68	165 g	8	5
Roggenbrot, Vogel's	59	30 g	14	8
Roll (bread), Kaiser	73	30 g	16	12
Roll-Ups®, processed fruit snack	99	30 g	25	24
Romano beans	46	150 g	18	8
Rye bread, wholemeal	58*	30 g	14	8
Ryvita™ crackers	69	25 g	16	11
Salami	[0]	120 g	0	0
Salmon	0	150 g	0	0
Sao™, plain square crackers	70	25 g	17	12
Sausages, fried	28	100 g	3	1
Scones, plain, made from packet mix	92	25 g	9	8
Sebago potato, peeled, boiled 35 min	87	150 g	17	14
Semolina cooked	55*	150 g	11	6
Shellfish (prawns, crab, lobster etc)	[0]	120 g	0	0
Shortbread biscuits	64	25 g	16	10
Shredded Wheat, breakfast cereal	75*	30 g	20	15
Shredded Wheatmeal™ biscuits	62	25 g	18	11
Skittles®	70	50 g	45	32
Snack Right Fruit Slice, original, Arnott's	48	35 g	26	12
Snack Right Fruit Roll, spicy apple and sultana, Arnott's	45	35 g	25	11
So Natural™ soy milk, full-fat (3%), 120 mg calcium, Calciforte	36	250 ml	18	6
So Natural™ soy milk, reduced-fat (1.5%), 120 mg calcium, Light	44	250 ml	17	8
So Natural™ soy milk, full-fat (3%), 0 mg calcium, Original	44	250 ml	17	8

* Average

FOOD	GI	NOMINAL SERVE SIZE	AVAILABLE CARB PER SERVE	GL PER SERVE
So Natural™ soy smoothie drink, banana, 1% fat	30	250 ml	22	7
So Natural™ soy smoothie drink, chocolate hazelnut, 1% fat	34	250 ml	25	8
So Natural™ soy yoghurt, peach and mango, 2% fat, sugar	50	200 ml	26	13
Sourdough rye	48	30 g	12	6
Sourdough wheat	54	30 g	14	8
Soy milk, So Natural™ full-fat (3%), 120 mg calcium, Calciforte	36	250 ml	18	6
Soy milk, So Natural™ reduced-fat (1.5%), 120 mg calcium, Light	44	250 ml	17	8
Soy milk, So Natural™ full-fat (3%), 0 mg calcium, Original	44	250 ml	17	8
Soy smoothie drink, So Natural™ banana, 1% fat	30	250 ml	22	7
Soy smoothie drink, So Natural™ chocolate hazelnut, 1% fat	34	250 ml	25	8
Soy yoghurt, So Natural™ peach and mango, 2% fat, sugar	50	200 g	26	13
Soy beans, dried, boiled	18*	150 g	6	1
Soy beans, canned	14	150 g	6	1
Soy-Lin, Bürgen® kibbled soy (8%) and linseed (8%) bread	36	30 g	9	3
Spaghetti, gluten-free, rice and split pea, canned in tomato sauce	68	220 g	27	19
Spaghetti, white, boiled 5 minutes	38*	180 g	48	18
Spaghetti, wholemeal, boiled 5 minutes	37	180 g	42	16
Special K®, breakfast cereal	54	30 g	21	11

* Average

FOOD	GI	NOMINAL SERVE SIZE	AVAILABLE CARB PER SERVE	GL PER SERVE
Spirali pasta, durum wheat, white, boiled to al denté texture	43	180 g	44	19
Split pea and soy pasta shells, gluten-free	29	180 g	31	9
Split pea soup	60	250 ml	27	16
Split peas, yellow, boiled 20 min	32	150 g	19	6
Sponge cake, plain	46	63 g	36	17
Stoned Wheat Thins crackers	67	25 g	17	12
Strawberries, fresh	40	120 g	3	1
Strawberry jam, regular	51	30 g	20	10
Stuffing, bread	74	30 g	21	16
Sucrose	68*	10 g	10	7
Sultana Bran™, breakfast cereal	73	30 g	19	14
Sultanas	56	60 g	45	25
Sunbrown Quick™ rice, boiled	80	150 g	38	31
Sunflower and barley bread, (Riga)	57	30 g	11	6
Super Supreme pizza, pan (11.4% fat)	36	100 g	24	9
Super Supreme pizza, thin and crispy (13.2 % fat)	30	100 g	22	7
Sushi, salmon	48	100 g	36	17
Sustagen™ Hospital with extra fibre, drink made from powdered mix	33	250 ml	44	15
Sustagen™ drink, Dutch Chocolate	31	250 ml	41	13
Sustagen™ pudding, instant vanilla, made from powdered mix	27	250 ml	47	13
Sustagen Sport®, milk-based drink	43	250 ml	49	21
Sustain™, breakfast cereal	68	30 g	22	15
Sustain™ cereal bar	57	30 g	25	14
Swede, cooked	72	150 g	10	7

* Average

FOOD	GI	NOMINAL SERVE SIZE	AVAILABLE CARB PER SERVE	GL PER SERVE
Sweet corn, whole kernel, canned, drained	46	80 g	14	7
Sweet corn on the cob, boiled	48	80 g	16	8
Sweet potato, cooked	44	150 g	25	11
Sweetened condensed whole milk	61	50 g	28	17
Taco shells, cornmeal-based, baked	68	20 g	12	8
Tapioca, boiled with milk	81	250 ml	18	14
Tomato soup	38	250 ml	17	6
Tortellini, cheese, cooked	50	180 g	21	10
TRIM™ custard, reduced-fat	37	100 g	15	6
Tuna	[0]	120 g	0	0
Twisties™, cheese-flavoured, extruded snack, rice and corn	74	50 g	29	22
Twix® Bar, caramel	44	60 g	39	17
Ultra chocolate ice-cream, premium 15% fat (Sara Lee)	37	50 g	9	4
Vaalia™, reduced-fat apricot and mango yoghurt	26	200 g	30	8
Vaalia™, reduced-fat French vanilla yoghurt	26	200 g	10	3
Vaalia™, reduced fat tropical passionfruit yoghurt drink	38	200 ml	29	11
Vanilla cake made from packet mix with vanilla frosting	42	111 g	58	24
Vanilla pudding, instant, made from packet mix and whole milk	40	100 g	16	6
Vanilla wafers, 6 biscuits	77	25 g	18	14
Veal	[0]	120 g	0	0
Vermicelli, white, boiled	35	180 g	44	16

* Average

FOOD	GI	NOMINAL SERVE SIZE	AVAILABLE CARB PER SERVE	GL PER SERVE
Vita-Brits™, breakfast cereal	68	30 g	20	13
Vita Weat crispbread	55	35 g	26	14
Vitari, wild berry, non-dairy, frozen fruit dessert	59	100 ml	21	12
Vogel's Honey & Oats bread	55	30 g	14	7
Waffles	76	35 g	13	10
Water crackers	78	25 g	18	14
Watermelon, raw	76	195 g	10	7
Weis Mango Frutia™, low fat frozen fruit dessert	42	100 ml	23	10
Weet-Bix™, breakfast cereal	69	30 g	17	12
Wheat-bites™, breakfast cereal	72	30 g	25	18
White bread, wheat flour	70	30 g	14	10
Wholemeal bread, wheat flour	71*	30 g	12	9
Wild About Fruit Apple Juice, pure, clear, unsweetened	44	250 ml	30	13
Wild About Fruit Apple Juice, pure, cloudy, unsweetened	37	250 ml	28	10
Wild About Fruit Apple and mandarin juice	53	250 ml	29	15
Wild About Fruit Apple and mango juice	44	250 ml	27	12
Wonderwhite™ bread	80	30 g	14	11
Yam, peeled, boiled	37*	150 g	36	13
Yoghurt, diet, low fat, no added sugar, vanilla	23	200 g	13	3
Yoghurt, diet, low fat, no added sugar, (fruit)	24*	200 g	13	3
Yoghurt drink, Vaalia™, reduced-fat tropical passionfruit	38	200 ml	29	11

* Average

FOOD	GI	NOMINAL SERVE SIZE	AVAILABLE CARB PER SERVE	GL PER SERVE
Yoghurt, low fat, fruit with artificial sweetener	14	200 g	13	2
Yoghurt, low fat, fruit with sugar	33	200 g	31	10
Yoghurt, low fat (0.9%), wild strawberry	31	200 g	30	9
Yoghurt, low fat, sugar sweetened, strawberry, Yoplait	33	200 g	31	10
Yoghurt, no-fat, French vanilla, Vaalia, with sugar	40	150 g	27	10
Yoghurt, no-fat, Mango, Vaalia, with sugar	39	150 g	25	10
Yoghurt, no-fat, strawberry, sweetened, Yoplait	19	200 g	13	2
Yoghurt, no-fat, Strawberry, Vaalia, with sugar	38	150 g	22	8
Yoghurt, no-fat, Wildberry, Vaalia, with sugar	38	150 g	22	8
Yoplait BFast breakfast drink, honey banana malt	33	250 ml	27	9

* Average

Reading sources and references

Jenkins DJA, Wolever TMS, Taylor RH, et al. 'Glycemic index of foods: a physiological basis for carbohydrate exchange.' *American Journal of Clinical Nutrition* 1981;34: 362–6.

Salmeron J, Manson JE, Stampfer MJ, Colditz GA, Wing AL, Willet WC. 'Dietary fiber, glycemic load and risk of non-insulin-dependent diabetes mellitus in women.' *Journal of the American Medical Association* 1997;277: 472–77.

Salmeron J, Ascherio EB, Rimm GA, Colditz D, Spiegelman D, Jenkins DJ, Stampfer MJ, Wing AL, Willet WC. 'Dietary fiber, glycemic load and risk of NIDDM in men.' *Diabetes Care* 1997;20: 545–50.

Liu S, Stampfer MJ, Manson JE, Hu FB, Franz M, Hennekens CH, Willet WC. 'A prospective study of dietary glycaemic load and risk of myocardial infarction in women.' *The Federation of American Societies for Experimental Biology Journal* 1998;124: A260 (abstract#1517).

Frost G, Keogh B, Smith D, Akinsanya K, Leeds AR. 'The effect of low glycaemic carbohydrate on insulin and glucose response in vivo and in vitro in patients with coronary heart disease.' *Metabolism* 1995;45: 669–72.

Frost G, Keogh B, Smith D, Leeds AR. 'Differences in glucose uptake in adipocytes from patients with and without coronary heart disease.' *Diabetic Medicine* 1998;15: 1003–9.

Frost G, Trew G, Margara R, Leeds AR, Dornhorst A. 'Improvement in adipocyte insulin response to a low glycemic index diet in women at risk of cardiovascular disease.' *Metabolism* 1998;47: 1245–51.

Frost G, Leeds AR, Dore CJB, Madieros S, Brading SA, Dornhorst A. 'Glycaemic index as a determinant of serum high density lipoprotein.' *Lancet* 1999; 353: 1045–8.

Where to go for help and further information

Your doctor
Your local doctor is a good starting point to assess your risk of heart disease and help you minimise and manage your risk.

A dietitian
For nutritional advice we suggest you seek the service of a dietitian who can provide nutritional assessment and guidance on an appropriate diet. The glycemic index of foods is a part of dietitians' training, so all dietitians should be able to help you in applying the principles in this book, but some dietitians do specialise in certain areas. If you want specific advice on the glycemic index, check with the dietitian when booking. Dietitians are available in public hospitals and privately. Check for the letters APD after their name, which indicates that they are an accredited practising dietitian. For a list of dietitians in your area contact the Dietitians Association of Australia (DAA) or check in the Yellow Pages under 'Dietitians'.

The National Heart Foundation
The National Heart Foundation is a non-profit health organisation whose purpose is to improve the heart health of Australians and to reduce disability and death from heart and blood vessel disease. They provide information and education on all aspects of heart and blood vessel disease.

Enquiries: 1300 36 27 87. National office of the National Heart Foundation of Australia: Cnr Denison St & Geils Court, Deakin ACT 2600.

About the authors

Kaye Foster-Powell, is an accredited practising dietitian with extensive experience in diabetes management. A graduate of the University of Sydney (B.Sc., Master of Nutrition & Dietetics) she has conducted research into the glycemic index of foods and its practical applications over the last 15 years. Currently she is a dietitian with Wentworth Area Diabetes Services and provides consultancy on all aspects of the glycemic index.

Professor Jennie Brand-Miller is Professor of Human Nutrition in the Human Nutrition Unit, School of Molecular and Microbial Biosciences at the University of Sydney, and President of the Nutrition Society of Australia. She has taught postgraduate students of nutrition and dietetics at the University of Sydney for over 24 years and currently leads a team of 12 research scientists. Professor Brand-Miller was recently awarded a Clunies Ross National Science and Technology Medal for her work in championing a new approach to nutrition and the management of blood glucose.

Dr Anthony Leeds is Senior Lecturer in the Department of Nutrition & Dietetics at King's College, London. He graduated in medicine from the Middlesex Hospital Medical School, London, in 1971. He conducts research on carbohydrate and dietary fibre in relation to heart disease, obesity and diabetes, continues part-time medical practice and is a member of the European Association of Scientific Editors. He chairs the research ethics committee of King's College and in 1999 was elected a Fellow of the Institute of Biology.